A Lucky Life
Interrupted

A Lucky Life

 RANDOM HOUSE NEW YORK

TOM BROKAW

Interrupted

A Memoir of Hope

Published in the United States by Random House,
an imprint and division of Penguin Random House LLC, New York.

RANDOM HOUSE and the HOUSE colophon are
registered trademarks of Penguin Random House LLC.

ISBN 978-1-4000-6969-9
eBook ISBN 978-0-679-60466-2

Printed in the United States of America on acid-free paper

www.atrandom.com

246897531

FIRST EDITION

*This book is dedicated to
the next generation of our family,
our grandchildren:
Claire Vivian Fry, Meredith Lynne Fry,
Vivian Aranka Simon,
Charlotte Bird Simon, and
Archer Thomas Merritt Brokaw.*

*Five reasons to live long
and drink deeply from their love.*

Summer

In the seasons of life I have had more than my share of summers.

A long run of sunny days and adventurous nights filled with lucky stars, uninterrupted by great personal calamity, rewarding in ways I could not have imagined in those formative years on the Great Plains. Our eldest daughter, Jennifer, reflecting her training as an emergency room physician, was along for the ride, but she worried.

"Dad," she would say, "we've never had anything go really wrong in our family. I wonder if we could handle it."

We were about to find out.

In February 2013, I turned seventy-three, or, more accurately, blew through the birthday, ignoring the actuarial truths that I was now in a mortality zone defined by age. What, me? After all, I spent the beginning of the seventy-fourth year biking hard through Chile and Argentina with some contemporaries. In the spring, I had flown to Africa to report on Nelson Mandela's final days and to accompany my wife, Meredith, to Malawi, where she has worked with a women's cooperative to establish a thriving business producing canned tomatoes.

We finished up at a lodge in Zimbabwe, bumping through the bush on wildlife excursions and, for Meredith, morning horseback rides. I started the day with swimming exercises, hoping to relieve what had become a persistent lower back pain.

I attributed it to long plane rides and an active lifestyle. If it didn't get better I planned to see a renowned orthopedist when I returned to New York, a sports medicine doc who, over the years, had treated me for similar ailments after a summer of rock climbing, backpacking, trekking, long-distance running, and bushwhacking to remote mountain lakes.

Probably require some therapy, I thought, never considering it could be anything more than an overexercised back. The conceit of a long, lucky life is that bad things happen to others. Jennifer's cautionary line about whether we could handle misfortune was provocative, and yet it seemed more of a group therapy subject than reality in our family.

Not for the first time, I was wrong, but in early summer I had no idea what was to come. I was determined to work through the steady, nagging pain and spend July and August on the trout waters of Montana.

That New York orthopedist, who's a longtime friend and familiar with my physical activities, ordered a conventional spinal X ray and, after examining it, reported that apart from some expected thinning of a lower-level disc no major anomalies showed up. He recommended more morning stretching exercises and over-the-counter pain relievers.

I happily plunged into my fishing schedule but then, inexplicably, took two hard falls, one on a rocky passage across my Montana home stream and one while in a boat on the Missouri River. What the hell, I thought, is this what happens when you hit seventy-three?

The back pain continued, resisting what I hoped would be the therapeutic effects of more stretching, Tylenol, massages, and limited golf and biking.

Besides, we had more to worry about in our extended family. Jennifer called to report that her mother-in-law, Lynne Fry, had been hospitalized with acute abdominal pain. Jennifer and her husband, Allen Fry, a radiologist, were on a second honeymoon when they got the call, and Jennifer immediately said that it didn't look good. They arrived at the hospital to hear the diagnosis: Lynne had a massive tumor on her pancreas. Pancreatic cancer is particularly lethal. Three weeks later she was gone.

Lynne was seventy-five, a small-town school librarian who had moved to the San Francisco area to be near our shared granddaughters. Meredith and I had an easy relationship with Lynne and admired how she managed her life after the death of her husband. She became a competitive ballroom dancer and took cruises with a companion she met on the dance floor. Her life was as organized as a Dewey decimal system card file in a community library.

When pancreatic cancer struck she accepted it without a whine or a whimper. Her apartment, books, and personal effects were quickly put in order for family members. She checked into hospice with the help of Jennifer, who as a physician is working hard to raise awareness of making the right decisions, for emotional and financial reasons, at the end of life.

Pancreatic cancer is one of the few cancers that worried me as I passed into my seventies. It's a lightning strike. It hits without warning and almost always kills. I've had five friends die of it, quickly, including the *New York Times* columnist Bill Safire.

I saw him at a Washington event in March 2009, cheerful and full of pithy observations. By the end of September of that year he was dead.

Still, even with Lynne so close to our family, it was more of an abstraction than a reality. Yes, I know pancreatic cancer is a threat, but to someone else, right?

For all the attention cancer receives publicly, such as at Stand Up To Cancer events during the World Series, or when big tough NFL linemen show up in pink shoes to draw attention to breast cancer, my guess is that most of us duck it by thinking, Not me.

The numbers blow a big hole in those "not me" assumptions.

The American Cancer Society estimates that in 2015 1,658,370 new cancer cases will be diagnosed and that in the same year about 1,600 people will die from cancer-related conditions daily. Those are big numbers, but the encouraging news is that there's been a 20 percent drop in the death rate from cancer in the last twenty years as a result of a reduction in smoking, improved patient awareness, and giant leaps in treating almost all forms of the disease.

President Richard Nixon declared war on cancer in 1971, and while significant progress has been made, this is a war of incremental victories. As we live longer, the odds are greater that cancer in some form will strike some part of the human body.

Lynne Fry's death was so sudden and so well managed by her, Jennifer, and Allen that it seemed a long way from our lives. Nonetheless, if pancreatic cancer strikes one in seventy-eight men and women, why shouldn't I feel vulnerable? Denial is a strong if imperfect defense.

Meredith and I joined the Frys and friends in the family hometown, Claremore, Oklahoma, for the burial and to share memories of Lynne's role as a school librarian. Allen's father, a local legend as a high school athlete and, later, coach, had died a few years earlier.

In size and style, Claremore, the home of Will Rogers and the fifties singing star Patti Page, shared the DNA of our hometown in South Dakota. It was all so familiar, the talk of high school athletics, the struggle to keep Main Street a viable business district, and, most of all, the shared familial loss when someone is gone, however long he or she had been absent from the careworn neighborhoods.

It was a mix of melancholy and merriment as Allen gave us a tour of the town, showing off the library where his mother had worked and the school where his dad had coached. We had a large family dinner at a restaurant famous for its high-caloric-count dishes smothered in gravy and batter-fried everything. One of the big ol' boy patrons left with a stack of carryout cartons and a .45-caliber pistol strapped on his waist. Oklahoma has an open carry law.

If that happened in New York people would be diving under tables, but I'd spent so much time in the West I was not surprised.

Fifty years ago I fled small-town life as swiftly as I could for bright lights, big city. At age seventy-five I have an ever-greater appreciation of these communities, which, at the end, remember and honor where you began.

That realization was not a personal epiphany. I didn't walk the streets of Claremore thinking, My God, at my age I have to start thinking about when I die and where I end up. I've adopted the guideline of Warren Buffett's partner, Charlie Munger, who says, "I wanna know where I'll be when I die—so I never go there."

It did occur to Meredith and me that now we would be the sole grandparents for Claire and Meredith, Allen and Jennifer's daughters. We had talked some about our aging and the mortality realities that come with it, but our immediate and even long-distance plans were for living, not dying.

I was in good health, with the exception of that nagging backache, and felt the false sense of assurance of someone who'd had a long, uninterrupted run of personal and professional good fortune.

I had big plans for the summer and fall, including finishing an NBC News documentary on the fiftieth anniversary of the death of John F. Kennedy and another documentary on the making of the feature film *Unbroken*, based on the phenomenal bestselling book about the life of Louis "Louie" Zamperini; presenting a few lectures; and enjoying several hunting and fishing excursions.

When we arrived back in Montana, the pain was not as troublesome, but I arranged an appointment with another orthopedist, in Rochester, Minnesota, when I attended an August board meeting of the Mayo Clinic board of public trustees. I had no intention of slowing down, and I was confident the back pain was a minor blip on my radar screen.

When I was a boy running with an older crowd I wanted them to see me as a contemporary so I avoided birthdays. When my sixties arrived I shifted to another form of evasion. I failed to see the benefit of those life expectancy scales that keep percolating up as we live healthier lives with access to better medicine. That was never more clear than when, in my late sixties, a fitness doctor said one day, "There's no reason you can't make it into your mid-eighties."

Oh, really?

My mother died at ninety-two, and the last few years were a burden for her as her body began to break down. Still, she hung on, even while saying, in her no-nonsense way, "Don't worry about me, dear; I've lived long enough."

I seem to have inherited some of her cardiac strength and I guess I thought the nineties had a nice ring to them.

A year earlier some old high school pals, also now in their seventies, gathered in our hometown and I asked how many could remember a local male in his seventies when we were coming of age.

We could remember one. All the others died earlier. My father died at sixty-nine of a massive heart attack, and Meredith's father died at age sixty-eight of a ruptured aorta.

In early August I flew to Rochester for the Mayo board meeting and arranged an abbreviated physical, including that other orthopedic examination. The Mayo orthopedist came to the same conclusion as my New York friend: lower-back thinning of a disc, some arthritis, and the inescapable consequences of age. He arranged an appointment with an exercise therapist.

My primary care physician, Dr. Andrew Majka, an internist, thought we should do a blood check even though one nine months earlier had indicated no problems. Although he didn't share his initial thoughts with me, he worried I had a hematoma from those falls taken while fishing.

At 7:00 the morning of the blood test I repeated what was to become a familiar mantra: "Tom Brokaw, two six four oh." My name and birth date, so the nurses and technicians would know they had the right patient. In short order, four tubes of Brokaw O positive blood were on their way to the lab and then into my digital files. I had a post-test bagel on the run, a Starbucks grande cappuccino, skim milk, please, and hustled off to meet the therapist who had some exercises to help that pesky backache.

As I remember, I also had a few errands in the Rochester commercial district that borders the Mayo complex, a collection of shops to serve the thousand patients a day who pass through the clinic. On one corner, a small store with a window full of wigs for women who have lost their hair to cancer treatment. On another, a sprawling shoe store with everything from stylish dress loafers to orthopedic footwear. Barnes & Noble (since closed) occupied a vintage movie theater building, filling it with racks of books, electronic tablets, videos, and gifts.

In the past few years the mall and hotels have been brightened by lively cocktail lounges, coffee bars, and a first-rate seafood restaurant. Altogether, Rochester has the ambience of a prosperous small midwestern city, one of many in that middle part of America to which Scandinavian and northern European immigrants brought their dreams, their work ethic, and their faith.

An English-born physician, William Worrall Mayo, decided to establish a medical clinic here after duty as a doctor during the U.S. Dakota War of 1862 and the Civil War. His sons, Charles and William J., became physicians and joined him. As its reputation for excellence spread, the clinic developed a unique systems management program to coordinate the care of the ever larger number of patients showing up in Rochester. Simply put, the patient was placed at the center of the care network and all the physicians coordinated their treatment while constantly communicating with one another.

Common sense, right? Madly enough, too much of American healthcare ignores that simple formula, with each specialist concentrating only on his or her area of expertise without communicating with other physicians on the case. Additionally, the Mayo brothers converted the clinic into a nonprofit institution, putting themselves on a salary with the rest of the medical staff. That financial reengineering headed off the temptation to order procedures to generate fees. It was the beginning of a healthcare system unprecedented in its patient management, reach, and standing, so much so that the name Mayo has been a global brand in healthcare for a century and a half.

The pedestrian traffic in Rochester is a mix—clinic

employees, local residents, Mayo patients, some in wheelchairs accompanied by families, others shuffling along with somber expressions. It is not, however, a depressing tableau, as it retains that Minnesota-nice, heartland optimism and the certainty that help is just up the street.

Hovering over all of this is the Mayo complex, three Rochester hospitals and a mix of large buildings housing state-of-the-art medical technology, physicians' offices, operating rooms, laboratories for routine blood tests, and research facilities for what they hope will be breakthrough treatment for some medical mystery. It is an $8-billion-plus-a-year business, including Mayo clinics in Scottsdale, Arizona, and Jacksonville, Florida.

As a child of the region and for a while a part-time resident of Minnesota, I always feel at home. Well before I became a public trustee, I shared the midwestern pride in the Mayo Clinic as one of the world's great healthcare facilities, known for its expert, coordinated care and patient efficiency. Our family will always remember how they put my father back together after a lifetime of serious back injuries brought on by his career as an operator of heavy construction equipment. He was a man who didn't know his own strength: One of his boyhood friends remembers him lifting a V8 engine off a workbench with his muscles alone. He came home from surgery at the clinic and never had another day of difficulty, thanks to his physician and a tempered attitude about work.

On the Rochester mall, summer days are given over to folk artists and local restaurants that sell the house specialty from makeshift kitchens. I opted for a pulled pork barbecue sandwich and headed for my hotel room to prepare a report for fellow trustees on prospective new members for our board.

Shortly, I was summoned to the Gonda building on the Mayo Clinic campus. A new clock was ticking in my life and I didn't have a clue. In about thirty minutes I went from the illusion of being forever young to the reality that life has a way of choosing its own course.

Dr. Majka invited me into his Spartan, functional office, where he said his boss, Dr. Morie Gertz, would be joining us to go over some of the blood results from the morning tests. Dr. Gertz is chair of internal medicine at Mayo and a nationally recognized hematologist. During lunch, Dr. Majka had shared with him the differences between my morning blood count and one taken nine months earlier. Okay. Maybe a low white count, I thought, or a parasite collected on that recent trip to Africa.

Dr. Gertz, a brusque Chicagoan, entered and went right to the computer screen, his eyes flickering as he scrolled down the columns of numbers. As he called them out, it sounded like a math quiz to me.

"A spike in the M protein cells."

As he finished his play-by-play, he turned in my direction and uttered the phrase for which I was completely unprepared: "You have a malignancy."

Making no attempt to prepare me for what was coming, he plunged ahead, saying it appeared I had multiple myeloma, a cancer of the plasma cells in the bone marrow, adding, "You've known others who had this." Frank Reynolds, the ABC anchorman (so that's what he died of, I thought) and Geraldine Ferraro, the first woman to run for vice president of the United States. She lived with it for twelve years when the life expectancy was much shorter.

"It is treatable but not curable—yet. We are making progress. Fifty percent of the progress has been made in the last five years, and I want to review your record overnight to make sure we've got this right."

Life expectancy? "Statistically, five years, but you should beat that."

I appreciated his unconditional, straight-ahead style. As a scientist in a difficult discipline, hematology, he was a numbers guy. He might have been absent the day his medical school class took a seminar in "bedside manner," but that was not as much an issue for me as it may have been for others. As a journalist as well as a patient I was looking for facts, not cheerful obfuscation, so I welcomed the "just-the-facts" presentation. Fact: Multiple myeloma is an incurable cancer, but as Dr. Gertz said, so much progress has been made in treating it with drugs and stem cell transplants that it is becoming a chronic condition, no longer wedded to the five-year life span prognosis.

Dr. Majka, standing behind him, was quiet, but I could see the concern in his expression. When he was first assigned to me several years ago, I learned that he was born in Buffalo, New York, and grew up in the area, beloved home of my late colleague Tim Russert, the legendary *Meet the Press* host and Buffalo's leading cheerleader. When I mentioned that he said, "Oh, I know. The two worst things for Buffalo were losing Tim and wide right in ninety-one," the year the bad-luck Buffalo Bills lost the Super Bowl to the New York Giants on a missed field goal from twenty-nine yards out with just eight seconds left in the game.

Dr. Majka and I developed a bond from that moment on, also sharing a passion for pheasant hunting and fishing. He's an enthusiastic angler for walleye, the feisty and very tasty game fish of the upper Midwest. Fishing for walleye in Minnesota lakes is the upper Midwest equivalent of a religious pilgrimage.

No talk of hunting and fishing in this meeting, however. The quality of life during treatment? Uneven. Cause? Unknown.

I had often wondered how I would react to this kind of news. Don't we all.

Now I know. Family first.

Our family had just finished some estate planning and financial evaluations. My earning years might be greatly reduced, but there's enough to get through this and keep the family commitments. As a working-class kid who found success in a profession that paid some big numbers, I am always of two minds: Yes, we live very well and I like that. I don't want money to define who we are, but with this news I was happy to have its company.

I worried my Irish gene might kick in and I would tear up at the news—the maternal side of the family are Conleys, originally from County Mayo—but I was surprisingly focused on the practical questions, not the personal worries. I did not have an "Oh, my god, I'm gonna die" moment. Not one, somewhat to my surprise. I later did remember Bill Paley's lament in his nineties, "Do I HAVE to die?" Paley was used to having everything his way—CBS, great wealth, world-class art, women, power—so his question was understandable. I was more in the spirit of my friend Jim Harrison, the writer who manages to be at once gruffly verbose and quietly insightful. We're the same age, and in an essay on his mortality he wrote, "As I aged, I expected to think about death far more than I do," explaining that after some severe health issues he's determined to go out with a bang—writing harder, fishing harder, and treating three-a-day naps as a Buddhist Noble Truth. That was a truth I came to treasure.

There were those fleeting moments of wondering, Is this payback for having a good life, despite imperfect behavior and decisions from time to time? Retribution from whoever or whatever has the power I keep hearing those television preachers invoke?

Over the years friends have often referred to "Brokaw's lucky star." I'd have to reach them and say, "Turns out that star has a dimmer switch."

Those were the random thoughts that appeared and disappeared just as swiftly as I tried vainly to understand this alien invasion of my bone marrow. Life has built-in risk and reward rhythms and the human body, that complex construct of brain cells, blood cells, bones, organs, nerves, and dermatology, is a biological marvel until it turns on you, and if you give it enough time, it will—dammit.

I had more immediate concerns: how to tell Meredith, still in Montana, when I have more tests and a board meeting the next day. I have a script for JFK that needs work.

As Majka and Gertz left I kept plumbing my reaction. Did they just say I have a form of incurable cancer? There had been no advance signals that something was wrong, apart from that persistent back pain, which I attributed to the two falls I'd taken while fishing and the long airplane rides to and from Africa.

(At one point earlier in the year I had even consulted a Montana chiropractor highly regarded for dealing with cowboy and skier back issues. I suspected he'd be surprised to hear the real villain is cancer.)

It was a left brain–right brain exercise as I tried to work through the consequences of this startling and wholly unexpected news.

Left brain: I've got to get back to the hotel room and finish rewriting that documentary.

Right brain: C'mon, this doesn't happen to me. At NBC I am jokingly called Duncan the Wonder Horse for my ability to juggle many projects at once and still indulge my passion for the outdoors. Does this mean no pheasant hunting in South Dakota this fall? No bike trip to Australia in the spring?

At the time of the diagnosis I was, at seventy-three,

just short of the life expectancy of an American white male. That statistic has percolated up to almost seventy-six years.

Seventy-six for an American male was a number on an actuarial chart that includes men who are obese, smokers, and inheritors of deadly family genes. I took my guidance from more than a few friends still going strong in their eighties or even nineties. Life expectancy was not so much a measure of how long I had to live but, rather, what was still to be accomplished.

Is it too late to learn to sail solo? Play chess? Get a short story published?

Most of all, I've had a life rich in personal and professional rewards beyond what should be anyone's even exaggerated expectations. I fully expect it to go on not because I want to write more books or appear on television more. I want more time with our family and in a contemplative, reflective environment. This will force the issue. Time to stop running for the plane and time to reorder priorities. Is that possible given the momentum of my life up to this point? I'll have some help from the next generation.

The Brokaw grandchildren bring all of that into sharp focus. Two teenage girls, two elementary school girls, and a new addition: a boy, born recently to our youngest, who picked out a sperm donor and delivered an irresistible child perfectly reflecting his American and Chinese ancestry.

As parents we are so consumed with the new experience of first having and then raising children, we often miss or rush through their unique stages of development. As grandparents we have the time and the eye for appreciating their physical, intellectual, and personality changes.

I don't want to give up my front-row seat for one of life's most rewarding experiences, the coming of age of Claire and Meredith, Vivian and Charlotte, and their prince, Archer.

In the meantime, Meredith: How do I break the news to her? We have been married for fifty-one years. I don't want to tell her on the telephone. I'll have to live with this for forty-eight hours and then deal with it when I return to the ranch. Not going to be easy.

As I made my way back to the hotel I kept checking my emotions. No "Why me, God?" I'm still a lucky guy. I have the best medical care. We caught it early. Unfairly or not, I have access to whatever resources I need.

I was a little surprised by the calmness I felt as I walked across one of the sky bridges connecting downtown Rochester and the hospital complex. In retrospect, it was a by-product of ignorance. For me, the diagnosis was at the beginning a bewildering intrusion that I didn't fully appreciate. I could not anticipate how completely cancer would take over my life, how my body and psyche would change. It was already attacking my healthy cells and bones, drilling a hole in my right pelvis, but apart from that persistent backache I had no physical sense of the gravity of the situation. It seemed somehow abstract, a series of numbers on a computer screen unrelated to my anatomy.

I stumbled emotionally for a moment. That morning a young IBM representative had interrupted my coffee to share his memories of growing up in Yankton, my hometown. His father had worked for my dad on a large dam outside of town, building and maintaining recreation areas. He said, "In our family we thought your parents were simply the best," adding with a laugh, "I delivered the newspaper to their house and your mother was always completely paid up."

Mother and Dad are both gone, but their reputation and legacy live on.

Dr. Majka called to confirm the next morning's appointment and to say, "I have to tell you I came home and spent a lot of time reviewing how we reached the diagnosis. I couldn't believe this has happened to you."

He wasn't foretelling my death. He simply projected how my adventurous life would be curtailed. I was touched but told him I was handling it well and appreciated his early detective work that led to the diagnosis.

Later, Dr. Gertz said, "Andy is the best. He's an internal medicine guy and there's a thousand ways he could have read those blood numbers but he nailed it."

Andrew, always modest, explained to me that the greatest challenge for a physician is what he calls "evidence-based medicine," EBM, in which a physician relies on a large body of statistics. Instead, he says, let the evidence presented by the patient sitting before you lead you to a conclusion, and resist a diagnosis based primarily on a mass of numbers.

Although at first he thought I had an internal hematoma from the falls while fishing, he kept connecting the dots and had come to the conclusion that it was multiple myeloma. Without his timely analysis I would have returned to Montana, still complaining of back pain brought on by two compression fractures in my lower back, beyond the scope of a conventional X ray.

I've now talked to two prominent physicians who have MM but whose diagnoses were delayed because they interpreted their back pain as the result of aging athleticism. Their orthopedists agreed. Months went by before they got the blood profile that confirmed the real villain.

Dr. Jo A. Hannafin, a top surgeon and director of orthopedic research at the Hospital for Special Surgery in New York, knew instantly she might be an MM victim. During surgery she lowered her head and felt a bone snap in her neck.

It could not have been that she was out of shape. In addition to her MD and PhD she is the first woman elected president of the American Orthopaedic Society for Sports Medicine, testimony to her wide-ranging research on athletic injuries, her skills in the operating room, and her record as a three-time national rowing champion.

MM is a low-population cancer, according to the official statistics, but I told Dr. Hannafin that I kept running into people—mostly male—who shared the condition. One MM patient even showed up in the outdoor plaza when I was doing the *Today* show with a sign: "Mr. Brokaw—I have multiple myeloma, too." We talked about our common condition and different treatments.

"When I was a resident," Dr. Hannafin told me, "if someone came in with compression fractures in their bones it was likely an African American male in their sixties. Now it is often a male or female up and down the age scale."

She was diagnosed about four months earlier than I and elected to have a stem cell transplant when drugs alone didn't get her numbers back to normal. It was not

easy. She was in the hospital seventeen days and confined to her home for weeks, battling fatigue and weight
gain, a new experience for this world-class athlete.

Now she's back to her old regimen, bicycling 162
miles in two days for an MM research benefit. "Finishing that was quite emotional," she said, adding, "I only
think about myeloma when I can't do what I used to take
for granted." I am silently determined to match her bike
ride at the same stage in my recovery.

As a physician, Hannafin thinks she's a better com-
municator now that she's had both experiences, those of
healer and patient. "I write down a lot more for patients
than I did in the past."

Dr. Hannafin's experience as a patient and as a physician is not unusual for cancer victims. Cancer of whatever flavor triggers a reflective gene: Just let me live and
I will learn to be a better person. In the past when I'd be
at an event for cancer research and cancer survivors
were asked to stand I'd be surprised by how many were
in the room, but there my curiosity would end. Now
when I meet a cancer survivor I want to know, "What
kind? Where were you treated? How has your life
changed?"

It is a club, a bond built on survival and the common
anxiety of having your body turn on you in such a vicious
way.

This was all new to me that humid Minnesota Thursday night in August. I wasn't in denial, but neither was I fully comprehending the radical change about to descend on me.

I decided the JFK script would be the best distraction and so I skipped the regular Thursday night board dinner and went to the computer, dividing my attention between "What do we know about Kennedy now that we didn't know then?" and "Does this mean radiation or chemo? Rochester, or can I be treated in New York?"

I needed to know more about this alien invasion of bone marrow. Google "multiple myeloma" and there it is: Plasma cells that help you fight infections become cancerous and multiply at dangerous rates, affecting bone strength, kidney function, energy. In short, in multiple myeloma good blood cells become bad cells and no one yet knows why.

The median age for onset is sixty-five. Men are more susceptible than women and African Americans are twice as likely as whites to get the disease.

It represents a small part of the cancer universe, affecting only about 1 percent of the people who get the disease.

That's as much as I wanted to know that night. I needed to get some sleep, and the more I knew about my new condition, the smaller the chance I would rest easy.

I wouldn't find a cure or even much more relief in the Google universe. There will be more questions, many more, tomorrow and beyond.

The phone rang. A fellow trustee and friend so close we might as well be brothers called to ask, "Where are you? Is something up?"

Ron Olson, the uberlawyer for Warren Buffett and various major corporate interests, intuitively knew that my absence from the trustees' dinner meant something was amiss.

I said, "Meet downstairs for a martini." Actually, we had one and a half as I explained what I knew. Since we share lifestyles, family values, physical activities, and, most of all, life stories, I could tell he was computing what this surprising, even shocking, news meant.

We both grew up in small midwestern towns, married very gifted local women, caught the brass ring in our professions, and never quite got over all the good fortune that came our way. I asked Ron to keep it to himself until I knew more. I did not want to become a photo on the Internet: Tom Brokaw, cancer victim. That was the beginning of a dual ordeal: how to find out more about the progress of the disease and settle on a treatment while keeping the news confined to family and a very few who would need to know.

I made it through the evening and the next morning's

board meeting, but I cannot say I was single-minded. As everyone left for the airport, I stayed behind for the mixed news from Dr. Gertz. He was right about the overall diagnosis, but his worries about the upper spine being involved were misplaced. It is multiple myeloma, he said, adding, "Eight years." I didn't blink but quickly asked, "Eight years and out?"

"Yes," he said, "but that's the current estimate for your condition. There's been great progress in treating this. We've learned fifty percent more than we knew before. People are living with this well beyond the estimates.

"We need a more complete look," he explained. "Do you have time for an MRI?" He wanted me to undergo the magnetic resonance imaging that requires full-body immersion in a high-tech cylinder.

I am told many patients are claustrophobically uncomfortable with MRIs. I usually like the isolation and the opportunity to nod off. Not this time. By late Friday afternoon the clinic is mostly deserted after a hectic five-day schedule, so I was alone with two pleasant technicians, encased for an hour with the eerie electronic sounds of the MRI tube, rehearsing what I would say to Meredith when I returned to Montana later that night.

Who else needs to know? Family, especially Jennifer, our physician daughter; NBC's senior management, my bosses. By the end of the hour my normal "bring it on" self-confidence was weakened a bit, not helped by the lonely, utterly clinical setting in which I found myself.

An MRI is a cacophony of weird electronic sounds echoing through a narrow steel tube as you slide back and forth slightly for a series of scans. Click. Buzz. What is it seeing? Are those rogue blood cells like the old Pac-Man monsters, eating up the good cells?

After an hour I had second thoughts about my ease with the procedure. It did give me time to think about my new life and how I might deal with it. As a journalist I immediately thought of keeping a journal, which led to this book, and the occasional reporter's notebook short-hand of MM for multiple myeloma.

Before the MRI I had scrambled to find a plane back to Montana. A usually reliable charter operator signed up and then fumbled the scheduling, so I would be getting home late and in a slower, uncomfortable prop aircraft. It was a long ride through the dark of a prairie night as we crossed out of Minnesota and into North Dakota before Montana was below. Big Sky country up on the northern latitudes, a muscular tapestry of geography still not completely tamed two hundred years after Lewis and Clark pushed through its mountains and rivers, the grasslands and forests, in search of a passage to the Pacific.

A midnight arrival at the small, deserted Livingston, Montana, airport was the beginning of the next difficult passage: when exactly to tell Meredith, who was waiting with another member of the family, our Labrador retriever, Red. A darkened car on a dangerous road was not a good place to break the news that would change her life as well. On the long eighteen-mile drive on a twisting gravel road to the ranch I kept up a steady stream of gossip from the Mayo board meeting and asked about some ranch issues.

In the small upstairs bedroom of our modest ranch house I made a drink—Scotch on the rocks—showered, sat on the edge of the bed, and said, "There's something I didn't tell you." I took her through the persistent back pain, the orthopedic optimism, and then the unexpected visit from Doctors Majka and Gertz.

"I have cancer. It's called multiple myeloma and it's a bone marrow disease. It is not curable but it is treatable, and they assure me great progress is being made."

I had rehearsed what I was going to say because I wanted to be precise but also because I was struggling to deal with that strange tug-of-war between a new reality and a way of life I couldn't quite believe was slipping away.

I said nothing about dying from it, because I don't expect to, but I said, "This will change our lives."

Meredith, always the cool and stoic family presence in times of stress, stared hard at this unexpected news. We hugged and I think I said, "I'm going to be okay. I've got you and the family but this won't be easy." Or if I didn't say that, I should have.

Still trying to process what she was hearing, Meredith asked about what to expect in treatment and a few questions about the exact nature of the disease, but we were both in a wilderness of uncertainty, caught between what little I had been told and a vast tract of the unknowable.

We've been together a half century and the relationship is deeply emotional, with a hardwired circuitry of midwestern steadiness to maintain the balance.

We fell asleep in each other's arms.

Oddly, the next morning my back pain had subsided considerably, so I drove two hundred miles to central Montana to join friends on a long-planned fishing trip, packing my lower back in ice. It was a special trip with Bernard "Lefty" Kreh, one of the world's great fly fishermen even at age eighty-eight.

The trip made no sense, coming as it did just forty-eight hours after my diagnosis and the ominous signs that the backache was more than an overexercised spine. While I had no inclination to tuck into a fetal position, paralyzed by fear of the unknown, packing my fly rods, waders, and assorted gear for a weekend as if nothing were amiss was equally foolish. By the second day I was a pretzel of pain, curled up on a friend's cabin porch, unable to gain my feet without a sharp passage of piercing, white-hot bolts through my nervous system. While keeping the full diagnosis from my companions, I decided I had to get home. Besides, Lefty was eager to meet my family and fish the Boulder River drainage.

If you need a distraction from unexpected and unpleasant realities on a long car ride, Lefty Kreh is matchless company. A veteran of the Battle of the Bulge, he returned to the United States after World War II to make his living as a master angler, trick sharpshooter, and columnist covering the outdoors. Along the way he became Ted Williams's favorite fishing companion, and for my generation, the word "legend" is completely inadequate.

On the drive we talked about his fishing trips with Fidel Castro and assorted other characters, and the sport we love. Lefty is famous for his aphorisms, having once said that one arrogant member of the fly-fishing fraternity had "as many friends as an alarm clock."

He never stops trying to improve on whatever is before him, from managing forty feet of fly line on a windy day to tying his shoes. But it is with a heavy, nine-foot saltwater fly rod in his eighty-eight-year-old hands that he becomes a maestro. The combination of rod, fly line, translucent leader, and imitation scuttling crab becomes a ballet under his light and unerring touch.

Lefty would stay at our place. I had arranged for him to fish with some local friends with whom I share a vintage dude ranch we've converted into a boys' fishing club. It wasn't difficult. Asking "Do you want to fish with Lefty Kreh?" is the angling equivalent of "Do you want Derek Jeter to help your son with his baseball skills?"

My back was not improving, so I was spending much of my time prone on our large upstairs bed, trying to anticipate which twitch would light up the pain meter. By nightfall I was all but immobilized, so getting out of bed was a roll onto the floor and a crawl to the bathroom. By the second day, Meredith called the Mayo team, and they began prescribing ever more powerful pain relievers. Nothing worked.

Our youngest daughter, Sarah, brought grandson Archer to my side for a quick kiss, and as I raised my head to receive it, my body exploded with pain. My knees involuntarily went to my chin and my arms flailed about.

Meredith said, "That's it; we're getting you on a plane to Rochester." By then I was in a haze of pain, agreeable to any suggestion that would relieve this cruel condition.

Months later Sarah quietly confessed that this was a terrifying passage for her, the first time she fully realized I would not be around forever, just as she was beginning this exciting new phase of her life as a mother.

Two highly efficient emergency medical technicians arrived with an ambulance from Livingston and a supply of Demerol. As one EMT injected me, the other unfolded the carrying chair that would get me down the narrow stairs and into the ambulance for the ride to Bozeman, sixty miles away.

There is a shorter route, but it is a back-beater in the best of times.

My new friends the EMTs were at once cowboy-tough and sensitive to my pain, confusion, and occasional hallucination. One EMT was my GPS system. "Okay, Tom, a rough stretch right ahead coming out of Big Timber." Or, "We're halfway home, heading up the grade west of Livingston." "Steady—railroad tracks ahead."

Prone on a stretcher, I was squeezed into a small jet with Meredith and two attendants from the charter company for the three-hour flight to Rochester. I was in and out of consciousness, so delusional that when we arrived in Minnesota I thought we were back in New York.

When I awoke the next morning in a hospital bed at Saint Marys, part of the Mayo complex, I was pumped through with painkillers and for the first time in forty-eight hours I had some relief. A new life was beginning to take shape, for better and for worse. There wouldn't be many easy days, but I was in a world-class hospital with my wife and had constant attention from the medical team. I was not in a helicopter in Iraq or Afghanistan, missing a leg or more, being rushed to a surgery station and an uncertain fate.

Having spent time at Walter Reed and many VA facilities, watching young men and women trying to put their lives and bodies back together, offers a perspective that came back to me again and again in the weeks ahead. Some of those visits had unexpectedly laughable conclusions. A few years ago former U.S. senator Bob Kerrey and I made a joint appearance at a Nebraska-wide benefit in Omaha, where we both had a connection. After a successful evening the grateful sponsor offered to fly us to South Dakota, where I had arranged a weekend of pheasant hunting.

My South Dakota friends were mostly Republicans but they were eager to meet Kerrey, a Democrat, not because of his politics but because of his Vietnam heroism. As a Navy SEAL he earned the Medal of Honor and was gravely wounded, eventually losing a leg below the knee to amputation. He was an enthusiastic hunter on the tough terrain, not at all handicapped by his right-leg prosthesis, but he wasn't much of a shot. No one commented on the misses and we all cheered when, on the final day, at the final hour, he knocked down one of the big birds.

As it happened, the following week I was scheduled to visit Walter Reed, and the chief of orthopedic surgery called to say he had a tough one. He would be amputating the leg of a young soldier early on the morning of my visit, and the young man insisted on meeting me. The doctor warned me that his patient would be heavily sedated and normally he would allow no visitors, but the young man was angrily insistent. So I went to his bedside, squeezed his hand, introduced myself, and said, "I've just spent a weekend hunting with a Navy SEAL who lost a leg in Vietnam and I couldn't keep up with him across the fields and over the fences, so there's a life out there for you. Thank you for this sacrifice and for serving our country." He gave me a small smile through his sedated haze and squeezed my hand back.

Struggling not to choke up, I left his room and the doctor said, "That was perfect. I have some other patients for you to see." So I made the rounds and then called Kerrey to thank him for getting me through the morning with the story of his life.

There was a pause and then Kerrey, lowering his voice, said, "You didn't tell them I couldn't hit my ass hunting, did you?"

There were other reminders from the new war zones. Leaving Baghdad for a flight home a few years ago, I caught a hop on a medivac plane to Germany. The attendant in the cargo hold, which was filled with wounded vets in various stages of difficulty, asked if I would pose for some pictures.

Of course. We chatted awhile and I asked if she had a family.

Yes, back home in North Carolina. Your husband taking care of the kids? No, he's up in the cockpit flying this plane. The kids are with their grandparents.

No whining, no "this is not fair." She and her husband had volunteered for the reserves and knew this day might come. They were part of the just 1 percent of our population to put on uniforms and fight our wars. Nothing is asked of the rest of us.

It is manifestly not right, and for all of the attention returning veterans are now getting, the fundamental issue remains: When we go to war, spending what politicians like to call "our precious blood and treasure," most of us stay home and are not required to change our lives, spending our treasure on ourselves.

As I discovered during my Mayo stay, there is more than some similarity between those who wear military uniforms and those who staff our big healthcare centers. Healthcare workers are not being shot at, obviously, but they are exposed to dangerous diseases; they lead unconventional, all-hours lives; they are mission-oriented and they work in a hierarchical environment, with the physicians on top and orderlies doing the grunt work at the bottom.

Twice a day I met with the medical team for a briefing on what came next: chemotherapy in a pill called Revlimid, developed from thalidomide, the drug banned in the sixties when it was found to cause birth defects in women being treated for morning sickness. For someone who had been taking only a baby aspirin and a cholesterol drug, my life was about to be divided by two pillboxes, one morning and one night. Within a few weeks I was taking seventeen pills a day.

Drug therapy for MM is advancing rapidly. There are two primary chemo treatments, and I was told that they were being constantly reengineered to make them even more effective. They have their work cut out: MM is a complex cancer, as all are, but this one has a daunting entry in any medical reference book. Myeloma as a description has its origins with the Greek medical genius Hippocrates, who did the earliest known work on cancer, which he called *karkinoma* (carcinoma) because the tumors often resembled a crab, *karkinos* in ancient Greek.

In modern descriptions, the condition is complex and treacherous: Plasma cells in the bone marrow become malignant and produce tumors, causing destruction of the bone and resulting in pathologic fracture and pain. A secretory form of the disease is characterized by the presence of Bence-Jones protein, a monoclonal immunoglobulin, which can cause anemia and kidney disease (and which explains why I am spending so much time peeing in a bottle for testing).

Somehow, and for reasons no one knows, my plasma cells went nuts and decided to attack my system, probably starting in the right pelvis area. I did immediately experience the bone destruction with the two compression fractures and more to come, but acute anemia and kidney issues were not on the screen. It was not a light pass, however. Jennifer later said, "Dad, your blood was sixty percent involved with myeloma."

Meredith was at my side throughout, emotionally attentive to me, all business with the medical staff and in the cockpit of the Brokaw command center, making arrangements for what was next.

At a dinner on our fiftieth wedding anniversary I said of Meredith, "I can have a terrible day and a restless night but when I awake in the morning and turn to her, she gives off that beatific smile and I know everything is going to be okay." I've been in awe of her organizational skills and cool efficiency since we first met, as sophomores in high school. Now here she was, more than half a century later, clicking off the names of the drugs and the dosages from memory by the second day, double-checking the refill compartments to be sure I was getting what I needed when I needed it.

Jennifer arrived from San Francisco and immediately joined the Mayo team as daughter, physician, and interpreter of medical terminology. As she leaned over Dr. Gertz's shoulder, reading my charts off the computer screen, I thought of how proud Meredith's father would have been.

When Jennifer was twelve or so and visiting her grandparents in South Dakota her grandfather, Merritt Auld, known to all as "Doc," said to her one morning, "C'mon, you're going to do rounds with me." At the end of their hospital visit he said, "Jennifer, you're our next doctor," one of eight in the family. He read her perfectly. Insatiably curious about the human body, with a built-in compassion gene and a take-charge personality, she is wired for medicine. She was just the team member I would need going forward.

Here in Rochester she fit right in, and I was learning a lesson in cancer care. It is important to have someone you trust to help manage the case. Jennifer knew what questions to ask, how to interpret the lingo, where to go for the latest reliable information on this cancer. I now use her as a model for others who develop cancer. "Get a Jennifer," I say, "a physician who is not on the clinical staff, a friend, who can be your ombudsman."

By the end of my Rochester stay Dr. Gertz had seen enough of Meredith and Jennifer to know he wasn't just handing me off to experts in New York. He was plainly impressed with Team Brokaw, telling me, "You're in better shape than most patients; you've got these two and they'll be very helpful."

These are the trials that test a family and define the character of the individual members. Having lived with four women—Meredith, Jennifer, Sarah, and our middle daughter, Andrea—for more than forty years now, I am endlessly intrigued by their distinctive strengths, interests, and instincts. In the weeks ahead I would need the combine they represented as each played a distinctive role.

First, however, the Brokaw pharmacy had to be opened and managed. Two daily doses of Revlimid, the chemotherapy pill, for four weeks, a break and then a resumption for two more cycles. Stool softeners for the expected constipation, an antifungus drug for my stomach, another for mouth sores, an aspirin, the cholesterol drug, vitamin supplements, dexamethasone (a steroid), and testosterone patches. OxyContin, the well-known pain reliever, at my discretion.

It is all very expensive. One Revlimid pill alone is

more than $500 and they're not easy to acquire. Only seven pharmacies in the country ship the powerful drug, and to become a customer requires a detailed background check and hospital authorization. Thanks to my General Electric healthcare plan for senior employees, my co-pay was just $15 per pill. What, I thought, does a farmer in Kansas do, or a small business owner in Kentucky, or any other multiple myeloma patient, to get on the list and pay for what appears to be, if not a breakthrough, at least a big step in the right direction?

With the Mayo team, we had decided my case would be transferred to Memorial Sloan Kettering, the world-famous cancer treatment center in New York. Dr. Gertz was very high on a young Sloan specialist who was compiling an impressive record in treating myeloma. Her name is Heather Landau, and she is a stylish, intense New Yorker. MM is her specialty. For the initial meeting she brought in a Sloan physician who concentrates on pain management. Dr. Roma Tickoo wears a white smock with the phrase "Pain and Palliative Care" in bold letters.

Given her unusual name I decided to just call her "Dr. Pain" but she laughingly rejected that, saying, "No, I want to be Dr. Palliative," making it clear that relief from the pain in my deteriorating bones was a high priority.

Dr. Landau agreed. "We think of pain pills as vitamin

P," she said. "We've had no cases of addiction and you'll want to be comfortable."

Other Sloan physicians and executives dropped by during the initial consultation, just to say hello and offer their assurance I was in good hands and would be doing much better by spring. That was comforting but in fact I didn't yet know all the steps to spring.

One of the visitors was a Dartmouth medical school classmate and very close friend of our daughter Jennifer and her MD husband, radiologist Allen Fry. Pete Allen, a former U.S. Army surgeon in Iraq and former Harvard football player, is now a top cancer surgeon at Sloan. It gave me an emotional jolt just seeing Pete, an offensive lineman for the Crimson, fill out his operating room scrubs. What he faces every day, the skills he's developed while retaining his droll sense of humor and his affection for Jen and Allen, add up to the qualities you want in every extended family member. These are people you'd like to keep around forever.

In shifting from Mayo in Minnesota to Sloan in New York, it helped to know the cultural geography of both places. In Rochester many of the accents have a faint hint of the dialogue from the film *Fargo*, and the Mayo drivers are often big, beefy guys who grew up on nearby dairy farms until that business became too difficult. One of my Mayo overnight nurses was a high-energy, athletic young woman who commuted an hour each way from a small town in Iowa to work weekends. When I asked why, she explained that her husband was the girls' basketball coach back home, the Iowa equivalent of being in the Main Street spotlight night and day. She wanted to be there for him during the week, when, in addition to all his other pressures, he taught fourth grade, and this year the class included their son and all his pals.

We talked about the prospects for the Green Devils and life in Osage, their hometown. She was surprised that I knew it was a county seat—from my days of working in nearby rock quarries during the summer of 1957. It was hard work, I explained, but I made the same commute to Rochester on weekends to court a nurse who wisely was more interested in her career than in my attention.

I think of my new Osage friend often—her nursing skills and, more important, the commitment she and her husband have to their marriage, their family, and their community. Those same core values are on display at Sloan, but they come with different accents and in a different setting. Sloan Kettering is a cancer treatment center exclusively, so I always wonder as I pass patients, What's going on in *their* bodies?

Is that cancer curable or just treatable?

Memorial Sloan Kettering is on the Upper East Side

of New York, a few blocks from the East River, and it is an urban intersection of modern medicine and technology, all directed at the treatment of cancer in its many forms. Walking the corridors of MSK, as Sloan is known to regulars, from one test to another, can be an emotional experience. A young mother, leaning over a gurney, whispering to a bald child, while Dad sits stoically nearby. I thought of our grandchildren and how devastating it would be to have one of them, bald and frightened, on that gurney. The emotional and financial turmoil, the complete immersion of the family in the struggle to find relief, the utter unfairness of it all, adds up to a price no one should have to pay.

The MSK staff reflects the immigrant roots of New York. A Haitian technician takes my blood. My pain specialist is from India. A native of the Dominican Republic checks my blood pressure and other vital signs. An Argentine MD and her South Korean–American associate survey my veins for a possible stem cell harvest, the extraction of healthy blood to replace the bad cells. An Iranian American physician, trained originally in Tehran, removes some stitches. As the Argentina-born physician put it, "New York is a melting pot; Sloan Kettering is a puree."

Quickly I was into the attack on those renegade plasma cells with the daily drug cocktail.

It is a complex procedure, what to take when, and Meredith instantly became my accountant, enforcer, and quick-study expert, taking detailed notes as the physicians worked their way through the daily routine of a multiple myeloma patient. Dr. Landau outlined her game plan: a twice-daily diet of Revlimid as the primary chemo drug, bone strengtheners, testosterone supplements, calcium, vitamins, and, she said, "We'll be looking at a stem cell transplant sometime around December. You'll lose your hair. Is that a problem?" No, but others had warned me that stem cell transplants can be arduous because they require a protracted hospital and home stay in germ-free conditions.

A friend about the same age was in his fifth year of multiple myeloma drug maintenance and doing well on drugs alone. He elected to pass on a stem cell transplant, explaining that at our age it is a serious interruption when we don't have an excess of days and months to give up. When I shared his story with Dr. Gertz at Mayo he was dismissive, saying there are no clinical trials demonstrating that drugs are equal to the stem cell procedure, adding that one personal experience is not an acceptable standard.

Another MM patient, a medical school professor about our age, elected to undergo the transplant and for him it worked surprisingly well. He was hospitalized for ten days and shortly thereafter resumed a robust life-style.

These are the dilemmas for cancer patients. Who and what to believe? A particular treatment is not foolproof, or, as many medical experts remind us, it is not math, with a fixed and certain outcome.

Physically, I had almost no trouble with chemo side effects. Fatigue, yes, but an extra nap would neutralize that and I didn't fight the impulse to crash for a half hour midday. Somewhere along the way I read an article about chemo brain, the cerebral effect of chemo treatments. Ah, I thought, that's why my spelling skills aren't consistently accessible and my fact-retrieval synapses aren't firing in reliable fashion. I'd encounter a long-familiar word and just stare at my misspelling, unable to quickly put it in order (no, it wasn't the onset of dementia). Spell-check became a close companion. Recalling from memory a name or a title was another long reach, and when I offered "chemo brain" as an excuse my contemporaries would laugh and say, "Hey, I'm not on chemo and I'm in the same place."

On these occasions and others when news came of a contemporary's health issues, the first reaction was generally, "Aging sucks." Born in 1940, I am not a boomer, but the tailwinds of that generation swept through my age group as well and we became part of the "always young" cohort. Aging was not in the game plan.

Suddenly I am shuffling along, cane in hand, trying to process all that the medical experts say is going wrong in my body, losing muscle mass and staring at the pillbox of high-powered pharmaceuticals instead of a single-malt Scotch at day's end.

It is unsettling to realize just how much control I've lost over my body and, by extension, my normal take-charge attitude. Cancer is running my life, and although I am central to the efforts to first slow it and then drive it away, I feel more like a test tube than the man in the cockpit, hands on the controls.

The uncertainty of it all is an unwelcome companion, and so I control what I can. I am methodical in my daily regimen of drugs and rest, physical therapy and diet. As a lifelong optimist I am confident this will work out, but it is frustrating not to have a more active role than just as an intake system for drugs morning, noon, and night.

Fall

Through August, September, and October 2013 I kept up a false front for my friends, who were concerned by my appearance and struggle to walk. Meredith and I worked up a stock answer. "Tom has a bad back, two broken bones from falls while fishing"—mostly true—"but he's making progress and he's bored by the subject" (true).

For a time I used a cane and, in the privacy of our apartment, a walker. My weight dropped precipitously, from close to two hundred to one seventy-five in a month, despite Meredith's calorie-rich morning shakes, pizza lunches, and protein-rich dinners, and at least one glass of wine nightly. However, I rarely finished a full serving.

My usually robust appetite faded quickly, mentally and physically. Not much sounded good and it all tasted flat.

Until this set in, a martini, chilled and straight up, was irresistible. No more.

That only added to the concern of friends, who know me as an enthusiastic New York foodie. Still, we kept up the cover story. Bad back. Complicated. Going to take a while.

It was about this time, in early November, that I completed what I thought of as a journey to reality. All my other medical problems in life had a sell-by date. I knew when the broken ankle would heal, the time it would take to knock out a parasite picked up in the Middle East, when a bout with flu would end. Cancer has its own calendar and insidious rhythm. The very word— cancer—has no redeeming qualities. It is a dangerous and mysterious condition. Paul A. Marks, president emeritus of Memorial Sloan Kettering Cancer Center, is one of the world's leading authorities on cancer, and he's weary of the attempts to soft-pedal dealing with it. It is not a "mind over matter" disease, nor is it a disease that has succumbed to the declaration of war against it.

As Marks puts it in a useful, plain-language book entitled *On the Cancer Frontier,* "The truth, uncomfortable and inconvenient as it may be, is that medical science has never faced a more inscrutable, more mutable, or more ruthless adversary. It is a unique disease. Cancer is, in a way, the body's war on itself."

Having spent his adult life on the cutting edge of cancer research and treatment, Marks knows whereof he speaks when he says cancers use all of the blood cells' capabilities to defeat the treatments we throw at them. We can understand the unsettling power of cancer intellectually, but unless it is eating away at our bodies it is something that happens to someone else.

It was my constant companion, out of sight but never out of mind. Accustomed as I was to having control, I did not welcome the new reality. The Brokaw brio was diluted.

Several close pals were worried I was hiding something very serious. We were part of the circle of Nora Ephron, the essayist, playwright, screenwriter, director, social arbiter, and den mother for a range of friends uniformly in awe of and in love with her. When she kept her rare form of leukemia secret until the week she died we were at once bereft and acutely conscious of what we don't know about our closest friends. As I continued my "bad back" story I finally felt compelled to go a small step deeper with a persistent interrogator. "It's serious but I am not Nora," I told her.

I also thought of my friend and competitor Peter Jennings, who developed a persistent cough shortly after I left the anchor chair of *NBC Nightly News*. Peter and I first met when we were in our twenties and we remained friends through our respective ascents of the network news routes to the summit, the anchor chair.

Peter carried with him the élan of a foreign correspondent, which he was for many years in the Middle East and Europe. Dashing and just affected enough to be teased about his ascots, he was The Prince of what came to be known as The Big Three—Peter, Dan Rather, and me. As journalists we had no shortage of work: big stories such as 9/11, the Soviet Union imploding, China changing, wars in Iraq and Bosnia, Silicon Valley, Mandela, Reagan, Iran-contra, President Clinton and Monica, Princess Diana, the contested presidential election of 2000.

We all arrived in those chairs as working reporters and for the first time in the history of the form we were not anchored in place. Portable satellite stations meant we could go to the story, and so we did.

God, it was exciting and rewarding, worth the exhaustion and uncertainty of personal schedules. I suppose we all developed an attitude of invulnerability, jumping on and off helicopters and chartered jets, being summoned to the White House for presidential briefings, broadcasting from Desert Storm and Belgrade, Manila and Beijing, Moscow and Prague. So when the news began to leak in April 2005 that Peter might have lung cancer it seemed surreal. Peter? A very heavy smoker once but not for a while. Peter, who liked to call you "lad" and host evenings at Carnegie Hall, seemed somehow above lung cancer.

Less than four months later he was gone. I still have a hard time processing the swiftness and violence with which his cancer struck. He barely had time to say good-bye.

As for me, I could not simply disappear. New York is my home and I had unfinished work at NBC to complete. Then I remembered one of the most memorable chance encounters of my life.

It was April 1982, and I was returning to New York from South Dakota, where we had just buried my father. News of his death from a massive coronary came shortly before I was to begin a new NBC News evening broadcast with Roger Mudd, who had come to us from CBS when Dan Rather was picked to succeed Walter Cronkite. It was a chaotic time as I flew first to California, where Dad had died, and then on to South Dakota, where he would be buried. Now I was headed back to New York to begin the new broadcast.

At the Minneapolis airport the gate attendant said, "I'm going to put you next to David Niven so others won't bother him." As I took my seat I introduced myself and mentioned a mutual friend I knew he had seen recently. For his part, Niven was all you would expect: dashing in his ascot, charming in his manners, and every inch the English gentleman. He explained that he had been at the Mayo Clinic for some tests and then quickly moved on to stories of President Ronald Reagan and their mutual friend William F. Buckley, Jr.

Odd, I thought, I'm having trouble understanding him, David Niven, the very embodiment of a well-spoken English actor.

He noticed my confusion and said, "Well, dear boy, I must tell you I was diagnosed with amyotrophic lateral sclerosis."

My god, I thought, Lou Gehrig's disease. It's terminal.

Just as quickly, Niven said, "Nothing I can do about it so let's just have a nice chat the rest of the way." And so we did as I mostly listened to tales of Noël Coward, Gielgud, Vivien Leigh, Olivier, Caine, and Guinness. He was all I could have wanted from David Niven as a chance companion—charming, witty, and self-deprecating, the very characteristics that made him such a star on the big screen.

As we began our descent into LaGuardia he turned to me and said, "Can we keep my condition between us? I'd rather not have it known."

I pledged my secrecy and for the next year, as rumors floated that he was seriously ill, I stayed silent. When he died less than a year after our meeting his son Jamie called and wanted to take me to lunch. It was, he said, a request from his father. "Go find that young man and tell him how much I appreciated that he kept his promise."

Now I was dealing with my own secret, and although my condition was not as perilous as Niven's, I did not want to go on television and have everyone look for signs I had cancer. So Meredith and I kept up the "bad back" explanation, but at home we were dealing with more than a bad back. Multiple myeloma had taken over our lives. The heavy pill regimen twice a day, the search for calorie-rich meals as my appetite and taste buds faded, night sweats, the frustration of a season without end as no one knew for sure when I might get better.

Through mid-September 2013 I was so immobilized at night I'd have to awaken Meredith to help me relieve myself. She patiently held a hospital container, a plastic quart bottle with a crooked neck in which I urinated. It was all done so slowly and methodically, we gave it a ritualistic name: tai chi pee.

I experimented with various forms of rolling out of bed with a minimum of pain. One smooth motion, legs first, pushing off the headboard with my left arm and muscling my right arm as an anchor on the other side. On my feet I grabbed the cane and counted five steps to a nearby dresser and then ten more to the bathroom door. Every move had a choreography and a destination.

TOM BROKAW

When it seemed more than Meredith could handle, one night our son-in-law Charles came over and slept on the living room sofa as a voluntary attendant. We're close to his parents so it was not surprising the next morning when his mother called to make sure Charles, an accomplished lawyer and wonderful father in his late forties, had been helpful. Whatever their age we never stop being parents to our children.

By mid-October, gratefully, I was making steady progress. No more cane. I could get in and out of bed unassisted. As my mobility improved I widened my world. I walked a block to a coffee shop for a morning toasted bagel with eggs, cheese, and bacon. With my slower pace and a mindset cleared of almost everything but my health, I noticed that my routine powers of observation were more focused.

Some of those powers were peevish. That fat guy shuffling along, smoking and listing to one side, he sure as hell doesn't take care of himself and yet I got the cancer. It was irrational but I needed some kind of venting. Just outside our apartment a bus stop had a life-sized poster of the New England Patriots' hunky quarterback Tom Brady staring moodily into the camera as he advertised UGG boots. On cold Manhattan days, shuffling cautiously over the icy sidewalks, my back wrenched in pain, I'd look at him and say silently, "F—— you."

60

It was my therapeutic moment.

(Six months later I met Brady for the first time at the Preakness horse race in Baltimore. He's even more impressive in person, with his model's good looks, easy smile, and small posse of jock friends along for the ride. I told him the story of my morning greeting to his poster and drew a big laugh from Tom and his pals. Even as a Giants fan I was so impressed with his good nature I made a winning bet on the Patriots in the Super Bowl against the Seahawks.)

Slowing from my usual frenetic pace, I became more observant of routine surroundings. In our familiar neighborhood I noticed more detail in the storefronts along Madison Avenue. Stately limestone mansions on Seventy-eighth Street, once the homes of tobacco heiress Doris Duke and others in the very rich class of the early twentieth century, took on fresh form as I paused to ponder the enormous scale and imagine the original occupants rattling around inside.

One day, slowly walking up Lexington Avenue, a route I had often taken, hurrying from the Seventy-seventh Street subway stop to our apartment on Seventy-ninth Street, I was suddenly aware that coming from the other direction were three couples. They were randomly aligned one after the other, seemingly unrelated, and each seemed to represent distinctive Asian origins. I guessed the first was Korean, the second Vietnamese or Laotian, and the third Chinese.

In my healthy days I would have blown right by them, but now I spent the next block contemplating how the face of America had changed, even in immigrant-rich New York City, and how I had taken it for granted. On one three-block stretch of Lexington Avenue there are five Asian-owned and -operated cleaning, laundry, and tailoring shops. They are bracketed by a similar number of manicure salons, all staffed by South Koreans, Chinese, or other Asians. When we arrived in New York thirty years ago the ethnic mix for these kinds of services included more Greek and Jewish tailors. Manicures were confined to hairstyling shops.

Our neighborhood has been undergoing a dynamic small-business evolution and I had not noticed, until cancer arrived and forced me to slow down, take it in, and wonder: Thirty years from now, what, then, for this stretch of Lexington Avenue, which is shaking off its gritty, aged façade and replacing it with new energy and possibilities? Will some digital magazine be doing a story on a Korean immigrant who started here as a tailor and became a New York real estate tycoon, with his Harvard Business School graduate children as his partners?

Now as I walk by their small shops, seeing the proprietors and clerks bent over sewing machines or ironing shirts early and late, I give them a silent salute, knowing their hard work will pay off.

By November this new life was the norm. I was living with cancer and trying to beat it, or, as I put it in occasional chats with my shaving mirror, "You've got cancer. Get used to it."

Writing this journal/memoir was helpful. It was a quick and productive link to my life of not so long ago. I also had a commitment to Clear Channel (now called iHeartRadio) for a daily radio commentary called *An American Story*—think Paul Harvey but not as long, not as resonant, though maybe I'll get there.

Our daughter Andrea, as a contractor/consultant for apps with a musical base, is my conduit to the digital generation. During one of her drop-by visits with her West Side New York daughters, Vivian and Charlotte Bird, I enlisted her as an idea source for *An American Story* so I could keep pace with the new generation. She was invaluable, beginning with the new glossary that goes well beyond LOL. How about A2D—agree to disagree. Or P—parent is watching. PP—parent is no longer watching. I'm looking for shorthand for Parent Doesn't Have a Clue. Maybe it's PDHAC.

Vivian and Charlotte are known affectionately as The Hooligans, a pair of vivacious, energetic city kids with a lot to say at high volume. During one visit I explained to them the definition of decibels as a subtle way to remind them to keep it to a low roar. It must have worked. On their next visit, on a day when I wasn't feeling so perky, Vivian walked in and announced solemnly, "Tom, we'll keep the decibels down."

These are the moments when family is the best treatment. I was reminded of the almost tragic case of Kevin Pearce, an American snowboarder headed for the medal round of the Vancouver Winter Olympics when he suffered a traumatic head injury during training. He was treated first in Utah and then medivaced to a brain treatment center in Denver where he was joined by his three brothers, mother, and dad.

His father is Simon Pearce, the celebrated glass artisan, who, with his wife, Pia, raised their boys in a family compound in a bucolic corner of Vermont. The boys lived in a remodeled barn out back, which quickly became a training gym–cum–bedroom and boy cave.

When it seemed Kevin would recover from his head injury the family decided to share their story, so I flew to Denver with my producer Jack Felling to accommodate them. It was not just another sports tearjerker. Pia and Simon and their boys, Adam, Andrew, and David, who has Down syndrome, talked intelligently and movingly about the shared experience of near death for Kevin. One moment he seemed indestructible, the daring

Kevin, and the next he's being choppered with traumatic head injuries first to a Utah hospital and then to the highly regarded Craig Hospital in Denver, which specializes in severe neuro-rehabilitation.

The family wanted me to know that David patrolled the corridors of Kevin's hospital, collaring every physician who passed by, saying, "Kevin is my brother. You've got to save him." Adam, the brother closest to Kevin, pushed him hard during the recovery therapy, even as he admitted he didn't know how it would turn out. It was hard, he said, shaking his head slowly, to see his vital, daredevil brother staring blankly into the distance.

Kevin later admitted there were times when he hated his family during the long, grueling hours of therapy. He didn't fully appreciate the extent of his injuries and he wanted his old life back, now. He didn't get all of his motor skills back, but the recovery was sufficient for Kevin and his brothers to form a foundation called LoveYourBrain to help people with brain injuries. It was a long way from that Denver hospitalization when Pia, tucked into Simon's arms, said, "I didn't know whether we'd get a miracle." When Jack and I wrapped our shooting I called Dick Ebersol, the executive producer of NBC Sports Olympic coverage, and said, "This is a story about family that will resonate with everyone. I think it should go in prime time."

That's not an easy call, because the commitment is to

the Olympic events of the day, and that is the expectation of the audience. But Dick has a matchless eye for what connects and gave us a prime-time slot. I appeared with Bob Costas, NBC's All-Pro sports commentator, and, as I recall, I asked him not to preview it, because I wanted his first reaction to be on the air. Unusual for Bob, he was momentarily speechless, letting what we had just witnessed sink in.

The Pearces are the kind of people I have in mind when I am regularly asked about my most memorable interviews. Interrogators expect I'll respond, "Gorbachev, Reagan, Bobby Kennedy, Nelson Mandela, Margaret Thatcher, Golda Meir, Deng Xiaoping," or other defining leaders of our time. However, I am most deeply moved and remember the occasion with greatest clarity when the subject is the lone white physician living in and tending to the two or three thousand black people in a squatters' camp north of Cape Town, South Africa, or the brave Swiss nurse from the International Red Cross who provided me with a file of the "disappeared" peasant boys who had been grabbed by the junta during the El Salvador civil war.

These were the middle-of-the-action stories that I thought were important and perfectly cast for television because they brought the events visually, audibly, and emotionally into your homes and hearts. Reuven Frank, one of the founding fathers of NBC News, said it best: "Television news is a medium that can transmit the experience of a news event unlike any other." His unspoken caution to correspondents and producers: There are times to step aside and let the experience speak for itself.

For much of 2013 I had been working on a two-hour documentary on the fiftieth anniversary of the assassination of John F. Kennedy, and the unwelcome appearance of cancer was not helpful. Still, I was able to participate in the screening, editing, and writing of the project while keeping my condition from the rest of the team. As I kept up the "It's my back" cover story I picked the feel-good days to record my on-camera appearances and the narration.

A week before *Where Were You? The Day JFK Died* was scheduled to air I made the rounds promoting it: *Late Show with David Letterman, Daily Show with Jon Stewart, Morning Joe* on MSNBC, *Today,* and *NBC Nightly News with Brian Williams,* while still taking the daily dose of chemotherapy. It may have been an American television first.

Meredith and some on my medical team were worried that those appearances were risky, given the heavy drug diet I was on. I was not. I practiced walking across our living room so when I hit the *Letterman* stage I could be sure of my steadiness. On Jon Stewart's show I asked to be seated when introduced—"bad back, you know"—because I didn't want to risk the big step up to the set. It all went well because, as I reminded family and a few friends, "ego in my business is a powerful drug." It was also therapeutic, getting me back to what I've done for most of my life.

Letterman is a friend and I thought he should know, so I called the morning after my appearance. He was stunned and has been very attentive since then, calling to check up, suggest dinner, discuss our mutual concerns about the environment.

The JFK documentary was well received, especially a segment in which Marie Tippit, the widow of the Dallas policeman shot and killed by Lee Harvey Oswald shortly after Kennedy's murder, brought to the interview with her a letter on pale blue stationery that I immediately recognized as belonging to Jacqueline Kennedy. From time to time Mrs. Kennedy and I had exchanged notes on books we discovered. It all started when I sent her Cyra McFadden's hilarious send-up of flower child and aging hippie life in Marin County, just north of San Francisco.

Just one week after the deaths of their two husbands Mrs. Kennedy, then just thirty-four and deeply grieving, wrote this to Mrs. Tippit:

What can I say to you—my husband's death is responsible for you losing your husband. Wasn't one life enough to take on that day?

I lit a flame for Jack at Arlington that will burn forever. I consider it burns for your husband, too, and so will everyone else who ever sees it.

With my inexpressible sympathy,
Jacqueline Kennedy

Caroline Kennedy, a New York neighbor, had control over the letter since it had been written by her mother and Jacqueline had left instructions it was not to be released. After a few cordial conversations Caroline gave me permission to use the letter on air, understanding the historical importance and the admirable sentiment.

As a young man I was bedazzled by Jack Kennedy's personal style and his literary gifts, supplemented by the magical pen of Theodore Sorensen. As I grew older and we came to know more about his personal life and presidential policies, especially his initial reservations about the civil rights movement, his Vietnam policies, and his determination to assassinate Castro, I was much more tempered in my enthusiasm.

Indisputably, the Cuban missile crisis was his finest moment, and perhaps the lessons learned would have been a template for his second-term policies in Vietnam, but we'll never know. That imaginative management of what could have been a nuclear showdown occurred months before his murder in Dallas, and in a way it was his exit line, so it took a prominent place in the instant analysis of his presidency.

So much of political success is symbolic, and JFK brought to the White House a highly charged atmosphere that inspired a generation of America's young to step into the arena. His aura, even when I disagreed with him, made public service and Washington exciting, a destination for a young journalist and political junkie from South Dakota. Ironically, my big Washington assignment was as White House correspondent for NBC News in the last year of Richard Nixon's presidency. Watergate.

Nixon lost the White House to Kennedy in 1960 and the California governor's race in 1962. He seemed to be through as a national candidate until Kennedy's assassination and Lyndon Johnson's troubled presidency. Winning in 1968, he was reelected by a historic landslide in 1972 and then began a long, tortured journey of self-inflicted wounds to an ignominious end as the first president to resign from office, remembered for Watergate and Vietnam. This is the same President Nixon who wisely saw opening relations with China as a bold strategic move, opened nuclear arms talks with Moscow, established the Environmental Protection Agency, and started welfare reform. He will always be one of American history's most enigmatic figures.

Kennedy and Nixon shared wartime duty in the Pacific and there the similarity ended, except each man, for entirely different reasons, was denied a full term to which he had been elected. To many, Kennedy's legacy as a man who changed the essential DNA of the presidency is a secure pathway to enduring greatness. The enthusiasts stumble through the endless sexual affairs and drug injections for his aching back and Addison's disease.

For all of his cultivated press coverage, most of it adoring, there was much we didn't know. A hundred years from now, with the clarity of hindsight and critical judgment, we may be closer to a conclusion on his presidency. Certainly his lively, wealthy family has been involved in so many triumphs, tragedies, self-inflicted catastrophes, and dubious enterprises that it could constitute its own Shakespearean chapter on America.

As a patient with severe back pain I do wonder how JFK endured his, along with the nagging knowledge that Addison's remained a controlled but not conquered disease.

As for me, my pain became sufficiently manageable that I could keep some long-standing personal commitments. MD Anderson, the celebrated Houston cancer center, honored former secretary of state James Baker at a Washington, D.C., fund-raiser where he was interviewed onstage by one of my favorite colleagues, Bob Schieffer of CBS News. The organizers sent a private plane so I could emcee the evening at the Kennedy Center. I made a point of reminding the audience that I am on the Mayo board and that the great work of all these cancer treatment centers was not a contest but instead a common assault on our common foe: cancer. However, I did not disclose my own condition except to Baker and Schieffer, both of whom had had experiences with cancer. Bob and Pat Schieffer and Jim and Susan Baker have become close friends over the years, and I didn't want them to hear my news on the gossip circuit.

The Bakers and Brokaws have an annual quail-hunting outing with our wives and other friends, so I wanted Jim to know the goal was to get the cancer under control before the birds were out of season. Those kinds of plans kept me focused on the future and better times. Multiple myeloma was now as much a part of my consciousness as days of the week and news of the day.

Which raised other questions. Did I pay sufficient attention to friends when they had their own encounters with some form of this pernicious invader? It is so often a hidden disease and deeply personal, the failure of your body to defend you against its mysteries. I have learned that when friends and relatives have cancer you can be sympathetic but you cannot be truly empathetic until you have it yourself.

As word began to slowly spread about my condition I was again reminded that a life in journalism has many dividends, not the least of which are the colleagues with whom you share common interests. The *New York Times* columnist Tom Friedman offered to come to my home and brief me on his recent trip to the Middle East. Rick Atkinson, the definitive American military historian, reminded me of a lecture tour we would conduct in Normandy on the seventieth anniversary of the landing, saying he would keep my seat warm and my martini cold. David Remnick, editor of *The New Yorker,* lost a family member to multiple myeloma and brought to our friendship informed empathy and welcome discussions about writers, reporting, and literary trends.

Herbert Allen, of the legendary Wall Street family firm, is the patron of our global bicycle trips and a longtime friend. He scheduled evening walks, assessing my physical progress and reminding me of upcoming excursions. As he put it in his brotherly-love sort of way, "We don't miss you as much as we miss your stories." Herbert and the writer Tom McGuane, a Montana neighbor and friend, are my age, and I could read in their touchingly solicitous notes an unspoken line: If this could happen to Tom, am I next? Cancer is an unwelcome companion to the so-called golden years.

In or out of journalism I am drawn to those with an adventure gene that never runs down. Yvon Chouinard, who turned his genius for rock climbing and passion for surfing, mountaineering, and fly-fishing into Patagonia stores, the retail outfitting chain that made functional outdoor clothing fashionable, called to plot the years he figures we have left. We laughed at memories of close calls and excursions into remote corners of the planet in times gone by.

A New York financial whiz and big-time foodie called regularly with offers of home-cooked meals. An NBC colleague baked cookies for grandchildren visits.

Two friends who are cancer survivors kept track of my treatment and knew when to call and what questions to ask.

A high school pal became the Brokaw correspondent for two other buddies from those long-ago days.

Maureen Orth, the magazine journalist and Tim Russert's widow, closed each of her notes to me saying she was remembering me in her prayers. Personally, I'd drifted from a prayerful life, but I was deeply touched by friends who keep the faith in a quiet way and offered their prayers as well.

·   ·   ·

All of this attention reminded me of a conversation with a friend who had an aggressive form of breast cancer. I flashed back more than thirty years to a Sunday when I drove my new, fast car to the home of Marc and Maria Kusnetz in the Catskills. Marc and I were a team at NBC News, correspondent and producer, traveling the world to document the collapse of the Soviet Union, the release of Nelson Mandela in South Africa, and the contra wars in Central America. We had a professional and personal association as close and important as family, the white-bread boy from South Dakota and the wiry, kinetic hippie carryover from Queens and Columbia University. His wife had been battling breast cancer, and Marc and I had been involved in a frontal attack on all there was to know about the best treatment. Unfortunately, her cancer was advanced and she came from a family with a history of unhappy outcomes from breast cancer.

Following graduation from Columbia's esteemed journalism school Marc spent a year on the hippie trail of love, drugs, and adventure in India and the subcontinent before coming home and meeting Maria, a serene Italian American beauty, yin to his yang.

After giving their sons a spin through the mountain roads in my new car I invited just Maria to join me. We laughed hard and hung on as I accelerated through hairpin turns and tried to put her condition behind us. She was in remission so I asked how it was going. I'll never forget how she stared out the window and said in a low, even voice. "Okay, I guess, but I know it's still there, the cancer. I can *feel* it."

It was a time when cancer counselors were in a fuzzy, feel-good mode, urging patients to "imagine a little elf with a stiff brush, just scrubbing away those cancer cells." Maria knew better. She didn't feel a brush. She felt cancer. We sat silently for a while and then drove on. She was right. Within a few months, she was gone.

I can still hear Maria's voice. Now I think more about the years I've had that Maria and other cancer victims were denied. With my diagnosis I quickly adopted a new attitude about age and years.

Seventy-three turned to seventy-four and neither seems like just another number to me any longer. As the birthday years climb, so does the cancer risk graph. George Johnson, a former reporter at *The New York Times,* wrote a widely praised book called *The Cancer Chronicles,* and followed it in the Sunday *Times* with an article entitled "Why Everyone Seems to Have Cancer." It appeared five months into my case, a time during which I learned of three other friends with cancer, one of them a surrogate son in his midforties.

Johnson got to the heart of the matter quickly. While

cancer death rates are going down modestly, the death rates for the two other prominent killers—heart disease and stroke—have declined dramatically. From 1958 to 2011 death from heart disease dropped by 69 percent. Stroke death rates, down 79 percent. Cancer in the same period?

Off just 12 percent.

Why? In heart disease cases, Johnson points out, changes in diet, exercise, and drugs to control cholesterol have been enormously beneficial, and if they fail, there are the mechanical fixes: new valves or pacemakers, bypass surgery and stents.

Cancer death rates benefited from the crusade against smoking (a particularly lethal form for my generation; I've lost eleven friends or acquaintances to lung cancer), but after that, very few preventative measures to significantly reduce cancer have been successful.

Johnson describes cancer as "not so much a disease as a phenomenon, the result of a basic evolutionary compromise. As a body lives and grows, its cells are constantly dividing, copying their DNA—this vast genetic library—and bequeathing it to the daughter cells. They in turn pass it to their own progeny: copies of copies of copies. Along the way, errors inevitably occur. Some are caused by carcinogens but most are random misprints."

Cell mutation is a biological wonder but it is not perfect. Johnson describes how "every so often a certain combination will give an individual cell too much power. It begins to evolve independently of the rest of the body. . . . It grows into a cancerous tumor." He reminds us that age becomes the catalyst for cancer. "As people age their cells amass more potentially cancerous mutations. Given a long enough life, cancer will eventually kill you—unless you die first of something else."

The statistics have a kind of cold, abstract place in our lives until they land in our bodies or affect someone close to us. In the months following my diagnosis I learned of a young friend, practically a son, with stomach cancer. Another young man close to one of our daughters with multiple myeloma. An NBC colleague, same condition. I heard that a former NBC colleague, almost exactly my age, was quietly battling an aggressive form of prostate cancer.

The strong connection between cancer and aging is evident every day in the obituary section of any newspaper. Well before MM became my constant companion I was a regular patron of those pages for the lessons learned from the celebrated and ordinary lives they chronicled.

Reading the obituaries took on a new dimension. Previously I had looked first to see what kind of life the deceased had led, especially if they were in what I called the Greatest Generation, the men and women of World War II. Now I was more interested in age. Here's a guy who made it to eighty-five and died of prostate cancer. That's a full life. Whoops, here's another who died at seventy-two, his family said, of cancer-related causes.

In our family, that is too familiar, for we had begun to struggle with my middle brother's onset of dementia at the same time I was going through the multiple myeloma stages. Bill was seventy-one when something began to seem amiss. He had retired after mixed success in the restaurant and residential real estate business, and was living alone after three marriages and only episodically connected to our youngest brother, Mike, and me.

When my mother began to fail in California he made more trips from Denver to be with us, but there were unsettling signs. He'd miss a flight by three hours, tell the same stories from his U.S. Army days in Germany, and keep from us exactly where he was living and how. By the time of Mother's funeral back in South Dakota his conversations, memory, and elusiveness were noticeably more erratic. Dr. Jennifer said, "Bill needs help now. I'll fly to Denver, contrive some story, and get him to a gerontologist."

I contacted some financial advisers to evaluate his net worth and budget for housing. Through her careful stewardship Mother left a tidy estate of almost $400,000, and we elected to divide that between Bill and Mike, who had a comfortable retirement program from his long, satisfying career as a telephone systems installer and supervisor.

Bill had good reason to keep us from his apartment. He'd become a hoarder. The living space was impenetrable, stacked with unopened boxes of polo shirts, cross-country skis, books, DVDs, and family photos dating back to the early twentieth century. As an avid and skilled cook, he also had a restaurant's worth supply of cooking pots and other utensils.

One more American enterprise emerging from the reality of the population growing old: de-hoarders. A small band of retired schoolteachers, social workers, and moving van employees moved in and sweet-talked their way through Bill's resistance, all the while clearing out the floor-to-ceiling stuff he'd accumulated.

They helped him decide what was necessary for his new digs, a middle-income apartment in a gentrified early-twentieth-century neighborhood near downtown Denver. With the help of some friends and Mary, the smart, compassionate advocate we hired to look after Bill, he quickly made the place, which had two bedrooms, two baths, and an outside deck, into a homey nest.

During my visits he was eager to show off the living room, framed by an oaken dining table restored by our father, an old-fashioned oaken dry sink that served as a bookcase, and a flat-screen television that had been sitting in its original box for six years. It all added up to a new life but it was one that Bill would never know, for his condition deteriorated rapidly. Several months before my MM diagnosis I flew to Denver to join Jennifer on a second round of geriatrician visits.

I let Bill drive a short distance to a favorite diner and it was unsettling. He stayed in his lane and drove slowly but went around the same block twice. We went shopping for an iPad but it was clear he could never master it. It was heartbreaking to watch him panic when the clerk asked for his birthdate as the beginning of a password.

He didn't have a clue.

Similarly, he didn't seem to fully understand why we were at the office of the doctor, Donald Murphy, a genial Notre Dame graduate and native of Casper, Wyoming. He chatted with Bill about the Denver restaurant business, all the while scanning his psychiatric and dementia screening results.

"Bill," he asked, "what about some meds, some pills to help you with memory and stuff?"

"Nah, I don't believe in them," Bill, always the family contrarian, answered quickly. "Besides, I didn't like that psychiatrist [who had examined Bill earlier]."

"Hey, I get it," Dr. Murphy answered. "No pills."

Dr. Murphy pulled me into another office and said, "We know what's going on here. It's a steep decline."

I broke into tears. Bill was just two years younger than me but his life was light-years different. Broken marriages, failed business, a stubborn resistance to anyone who volunteered to help. Yet he was natively smart, a voracious reader and a public policy wonk. Earlier in his Denver stay I had introduced him to former governor Dick Lamm, and Lamm had said, "Bill actually knows about and cares about municipal transportation. And a lot of other issues under the radar."

In the family he was famously stubborn and outspoken after a childhood of painful shyness. As one of his stepsons put it, "There is the way everyone agrees on and then there is Bill's way."

We all worried that this stubbornness would make another move difficult, this one to an assisted living facility. Mary, the advocate, found a new facility in Lakewood, a well-organized three-floor home for seniors with the onset of dementia, the middle stage, and those who are deep, deep into the dreaded disease. It had all the perks of modern living: a coffee and snack bar, a well-appointed dining room, a small theater with a giant television screen, and small but comfortable apartments. The surrounding grounds were parklike, with recently planted trees and a lawn sloping down to a new development of suburban homes.

These facilities are a growth industry, with the number of deaths from Alzheimer's having increased 68 percent between the years 2000 and 2012. By 2025 the number of people age sixty-five and older with Alzheimer's is expected to climb another 40 percent, to more than seven million nationwide.

The stark numbers don't stop there. It is the sixth leading cause of death in the United States, the fifth leading cause of death for those sixty-five and older.

If a cure is not found, the cost of Alzheimer's is expected to soar to $1.2 trillion by 2050 from $203 billion in 2013. It will drive up the cost of the already overburdened Medicare and Medicaid by 500 percent in the same period.

When I visited Bill's prospective new home the lobby was filled with residents planning day excursions or summer bus trips to Mt. Rushmore, in South Dakota. One perky woman, about my age, gray-haired with a new permanent, said, "Say, you look familiar. Who are you?" I told her and she said, "Well, you have to come to my birthday party tomorrow. We're going to have fun." I said, "Oh, I am so sorry, I have to leave today." And then, plumbing for more information, I added, "You look so young. How old are you?" She shot me a stern look and said, "You think if I knew that I'd be in here?!?" And burst into laughter.

Bill could be happy here, I thought.

He moved without much complaining and it was another opportunity to clear out more of his accumulated stuff, including wine, cookware, and sporting goods equipment, most of which had not been used in a long time.

Dealing with dementia patients is a delicate dance for family members, caregivers, and the afflicted. It is one step compassion, two steps patience, three steps deception. After initial protests about discarding some personal belongings Bill quickly forgot he owned them, and by then they were out the door and on their way to the Salvation Army.

Earlier he gave up his car when Mary persuaded him it needed a complete inspection and then conspired with the dealer to load up the estimate of costs so it would be impractical for him to pay them. He reluctantly agreed to sell the car and relied instead on a livery service.

Bill's new home was part of a boom in assisted living facilities around the country, one more manifestation of our aging demographics. The staff was well trained and responsive to our inquiries and requests. He had a sunny one-bedroom apartment with a small kitchen. It was a good fit. It was also expensive. His housing, medical care, and association with the highly efficient Mary ran about $90,000 a year. We worked out a formula for Bill to pay his primary expenses from his inheritance and I picked up some incidentals, relieved I was in a position to help immediately and when Bill's nest egg ran out.

What about those families with modest resources or none at all? Grandma goes in the back bedroom or in a warehouselike facility. It's now estimated that five million people are living with dementia in America, and unless there is medical relief soon that number will grow steadily. The Alzheimer's Association estimates that more than fifteen million family members and friends give more than seventeen and a half billion hours of unpaid care to Alzheimer's patients annually. Medicare and Medicaid help but the financial and emotional price lands on the immediate family, most of them working or middle class and already struggling with their own daily cost of living.

By Thanksgiving Bill's condition had deteriorated and he had reached a stage at which he was irascible. He argued with everyone. Nothing made him happy, especially the meal service, an area where he claimed expertise, having been in the restaurant business for so long.

As a teenager we called him Prince William because he was fastidious about his wardrobe and appearance. Those days were gone as he refused to shower regularly, often sleeping in the same clothes for two or three nights at a time. He needed more supervision, so arrangements were made to move him into memory care, a section of the home where the guests are never out of sight of the attendants and their daily activities resemble a play group for grown-ups.

Mary took him out to lunch while the staff moved his essential belongings into a studio apartment, much smaller than his original space. Everyone was prepared for him to blow up when he realized the switch had been made but he barely noticed, one more sign of how rapidly his condition was deteriorating.

So much of Bill's bravado is a cover for what is a vulnerable and sweet personality. We see flashes of that when friends visit or during telephone calls when he remembers a long-gone pet dog or a recent photo of his nieces. Then he retreats into that private world of anger, forgetfulness, and disconnect from the orderliness the rest of us take for granted.

We're going through the trials and joy brought on by the journey of the modern American family. Our youngest daughter, Sarah, brought the joy when she decided to become a single mom at age forty-two after a long line of suitors failed to spark the necessary fire in her heart. The sperm donor pregnancy and birth after several tries was a tribute to imaginative new approaches to fertility and childbearing. The sperm donor, a close friend, pitched right in as a surrogate father, a comforting development to Meredith and me, separated as we were from Sarah and Archer by three thousand miles.

When cancer struck, Archer became even more important in my life because he gave me more reason to survive. I found myself thinking, "Well, if I make eight years Archer will be in the second grade and ready for his first fishing rod that summer."

When Sarah took Archer to see Uncle Bill in his new home it had not been a good week—until they arrived. Bill wept with joy when he saw Sarah and her son. As Sarah rolled the always smiling Archer through the dining room the other residents lit up and the staff asked Sarah, not entirely in jest, if she could bring him by once a week.

All these parts of our family were not on my radar screen a few years earlier. How do you plan ten years or even five years earlier for one six-month period in which you develop cancer and your brother is institutionalized with Alzheimer's? When those disconnected realities arrived we were fortified by strong family ties and an acute awareness of our need to become even more supportive of one another. We'd been through the onset of dementia with my mother and brother Mike's mother-in-law.

Any one of the conditions brings a unique challenge to a family. Given the trends in cancer, dementia, and aging, there are many families of our generation facing similar challenges. As healthcare costs continue to rise, or even if they level off and become more manageable under the plan President Obama struggled to put in place, the price tag for the middle and working class facing complex medical problems will continue to be a crushing burden. There are estimates that two-thirds of the family bankruptcies filed in America are the result of healthcare costs that could not be paid.

Moreover, the costs to the economy are their own form of cancer to society. If a manufacturer, small business, or giant retailer is spending an ever-larger percentage of their annual revenues on healthcare they look for the exits.

Below the middle class, there is another reality that cannot be sustained. If 20 percent of the American population is hovering at poverty levels because of the high cost of housing, healthcare, higher education, and the cultural pressures for more consumer goods, where do people turn, with so many states reluctant to fund Medicaid under the formula worked out in President Obama's Affordable Care Act, the national attempt to control healthcare costs?

At the end of the day, the objective reality of an aging population with its attendant health issues, the demands of a highly technical workplace, and the uneven results of public education are all strains on the American assumption of a level playing field. It is not just a dollars-and-cents issue. It is a commentary on our failure as a nation to adapt to the objective realities of profound change and how it affects the general welfare of our citizenry.

A few years ago I led a discussion on this subject before an audience of some of the most entrepreneurial, financially successful executives in the country. I asked how many knew how much they spent on their healthcare the prior year. Sheepishly, they came to me to say, "I haven't a clue." One said, "I wouldn't even know who to ask."

We're a nation of informed consumers when it comes to buying flat-screen TVs, automobiles, running shoes, supermarket specials, and gas at the pump—but healthcare? Not a clue. It's time for everyone to get involved. For example, the older members of my power audience were all Medicare-eligible and no doubt on the rolls. My guess is that the now-highlighted 1 percent crowd would be willing to pay more into Medicare and take less to make more room for the needs of the other 99 percent.

Some argue that this would turn Medicare into a segmented welfare program and divide the country even more. I don't buy it. It doesn't hold up against the long-term realities of the needs and costs.

The madness of one part of the American healthcare economy filled up an entire edition of *Time* magazine in February 2013. It was called "Bitter Pill: Why Medical Bills Are Killing Us," and it was by Steven Brill, a bulldog-tough investigative reporter who has turned the piece into a bestselling book, *America's Bitter Pill: Money, Politics, Backroom Deals, and the Fight to Fix Our Broken Healthcare System.*

Sloan and other high-end New York hospitals are world-class facilities competing for the best and brightest physicians and to keep their beds filled with patients. They are also now part of a healthcare delivery systems arms war. New York television screens are filled with slick, persuasive commercials featuring ordinary Americans who promote the virtues of a knee replacement surgery at the Hospital for Special Surgery and New York–Presbyterian's campaign of real patients appearing in black-and-white commercials describing their treatment.

One, featuring a nine-year-old girl sharing her story of complicated cancer surgery, and poignantly bungling the word "Presbyterian," has been viewed on YouTube more than seventy thousand times.

New York–area hospitals are spending more than $80 million annually on advertising, including stamping their names on subway cars and jitneys, and buying pop-ups on search engines and Google sites. Those expenditures, twinned with the acquisition of other healthcare systems, have turned the American hospital business into something resembling those nineteenth-century land rushes in California gold country or Texas and Oklahoma oil territory. Administrators and boards are authorizing huge acquisitions and marketing campaigns, crashing through doors and spending tons of cash in hopes they hit a mother lode or a gusher. In the uncertain political and economic environment of future healthcare it is a big gamble.

Cancercenter.com, a private treatment company, buys an hour of television time regularly for an infomercial that is as skillfully produced as any documentary on ESPN. Someone has to pay for all that expensive marketing, the executives who manage it and the star physicians who can deliver on the promise of those infomercials.

New York–area hospitals and healthcare systems and hospitals across the country have adopted catchy slogans in their campaigns to attract patients: HOPE LIVES HERE—AMAZING THINGS ARE HAPPENING HERE—ANY GIVEN MOMENT.

The vice president of marketing at New York–Presbyterian, David Feinberg, says, "We don't see it as an expense; we think of it as a strategic investment."

Brill takes readers through the hieroglyphics of billing patients. The codes and pricing rationale more closely resemble a Monty Python skit than a transparent financial transaction. Eighteen dollars for a diabetes test strip available at Walmart for fifty-five cents. A patient with what turned out to be severe heartburn was charged almost $200 for a drug test. She was sixty-four years old. If she had been sixty-five and on Medicare the bill for the test would have been $13.94.

Altogether, her heartburn trip to the hospital, including ambulance ride, doctors, hospital fees, and tests, came to $21,000, and she had no insurance. Who did pay? If you were a patient at that hospital and had insurance, you pitched in without knowing it.

Brill's investigation turned up one horror story after another along those lines, many much worse, an experience I encountered while producing two hour-long documentaries on healthcare costs in the eighties and nineties. How to change that? I decided that the front lines of medicine, the physicians, have to get deeply involved.

In the spring of 2013, before my MM diagnosis, I received an honorary degree from the Mayo Medical School and gave the commencement address to the hundred graduates, almost equally divided between men and women. I am in awe of the bandwidth—the brain power—it takes to become a physician, the dedication, the imagination and energy, the compassion, and, in the new generation, the greater commitment to a level playing field for the patient population. With all of that in mind, I began with a favorite anecdote from Dick Butkus, the legendary jackhammer-tough Chicago Bears linebacker.

When asked why his college major was physical education he said, "If I was smart enough to be a doctor, I'd be a doctor." I told the graduates I shared that with Butkus but that I did have some observations about patients and doctors, based on personal and professional experience:

As your commencement speaker I cannot tell you how to read a scan, crack a chest, set a bone, insert a stent, prescribe the right combination of drugs, or any of the other procedures you're about to take into the world.

What I can talk about is my own empirical observation on the state of healthcare and doctor-patient relationships.

To begin, you're headed off to your residencies at a time of considerable confusion and uncertainty in the construct of the delivery of and payment for healthcare in America.

That [cost and payment] system in its current form is unsustainable on a national level. It is too opaque, too chaotic, too expensive, too uneven, and too inefficient.

My best guess is that it will be fine-tuned—

with more state-by-state flexibility and more private economy variations.

But what will not change is that the delivery of healthcare cannot slow or stop while this is sorted out. We're attempting to change tires on a semi trailer truck while going eighty miles an hour.

That's where you come in.

I am persuaded that even with Google most patients enter a doctor's office or a hospital as if it were a Mayan temple, representing an ancient and mysterious culture with no language in common with the visitor.

Judgment is suspended and the visitor in his or her own mind takes on the character of an anatomical chart, a mute and inanimate object, worried about asking the dumb question or befuddled by the new terms they're hearing.

That separation from their world and your world is a reality that to one degree or another will affect your short- and long-term future.

As a physician you have special standing with those who are on the outside looking in—and a special understanding because you are on the inside looking out.

To return where I began, a high priority for your profession is to demystify the way medicine presents itself to the world.

As graduates of the Mayo system I am confident they understood that. The clinic is a patient-friendly system with expansive lobbies and sunny solariums as a welcome retreat for patients facing the unknown or a defined condition that has no good outcome.

The real genius is in the management of every patient who comes through the doors. A Saudi prince may get more personalized attention than a Wisconsin schoolteacher, but both will be the central figure in a system where all of the attending physicians and technicians on the case are sharing the same information and constantly communicating with one another about what's best for the patient. Sounds logical, no?

In too many healthcare facilities and in too many specialized practices the patient is a one-off: advised or treated and then passed along with no connecting communication between the last and next physician. One of the enduring lessons of my cancer experience is that of the need for a personal ombudsman, a physician not directly involved in the treatment but with broad knowledge so he or she can interpret the primary caregiver's approach. Jennifer did that for me and I would like to see an institutional approach to the need.

We could have retired physicians available at major healthcare systems to assist befuddled patients and their families through the maze. We should take a cue from our most successful American-made enterprise of the past twenty years: Silicon Valley, home of the entrepreneurial whiz kids who gave us first the portable computer and then a galaxy of applications that continue to change how we communicate, buy and sell, do research, entertain and be entertained. The digital world is our Big Bang.

And what's the driving motivation? Be disruptive. Challenge convention and change it positively.

We need to be disruptive in our approach to the obvious challenges of our time, one of which is healthcare. We have in this country great medical schools, physicians, researchers, healthcare systems, and pharmaceutical companies entangled in an imperfect system. President Obama's attempt to reform that was ambitious and in some states, notably Kentucky, it is working. However, from the beginning it was too complicated and too wide-ranging, leading to a series of exemptions and variations to satisfy states that wanted to tailor it for their unique needs and political realities.

The political perception was not helped when the president assured everyone they could keep the doctor they have, a promise he was forced to retract. While the Democrats fumbled the construct of the plan, Republicans were equally derelict in not presenting a comprehensive bill of their own. They chose to simply make it a political football, punting at every opportunity.

My own impression from the beginning was that it would have been more efficient to roll out reform in stages, beginning with a plan for just the uninsured and then forming medical, corporate, and political coalitions to resolve the remaining issues.

As 2013 came to a close I was in a cancer treatment rhythm. My life was ritualistic: a chemotherapy capsule and other pills in the morning, followed by physical therapy designed to arrest the deterioration of muscle tone and balance. At mealtime I had a slightly more robust appetite, but my calorie intake was probably two-thirds of what it had been prediagnosis.

That was not an ominous development until I slid past 175 pounds and couldn't turn the scale back up. So I forced more of the liquid nutritional supplements into my system and arrested the slide.

Weight loss was another reminder that other forces were controlling my body, and while I understood intellectually what was going on, I resented it.

When do I get some control back? I wondered.

Winter

By early December 2013 my new normal was due for another reality check. Were the drugs, especially Revlimid, working? To know, I had to undergo further testing, including a bone marrow extraction—a series of needle injections into my right pelvic area. It was neither a benign experience nor intolerable, if you can tolerate a sharp jab of pain followed by an electrical charge through the nervous system of the lower extremities.

The other two parts were a check of the blood chemistry and a PET scan, that nuclear medicine pinball machine, locating the bone deterioration. The results would help determine the next step. Specifically, would a stem cell transplant be necessary? There are clinical trials under way on the question of whether transplants can be set aside in favor of continuing just a drug assault on the myeloma. Some specialists are choosing that option before the trials are finished. Others are awaiting the outcome before going the drug-only route.

As I waited for the results of my tests and the choice that Dr. Landau would make, Nelson Mandela died in South Africa. The loss of this great man triggered so many memories. We first met in 1990, when he was released from prison after more than a quarter-century behind bars. Early that year, thanks to a tip from a friend in the South African government, I managed to get to Johannesburg before it was announced by the apartheid regime that Mandela would be freed.

For twenty-seven years he had been seen by very few in the outside world. Journalists relied on old, grainy black-and-white photographs of him as a young rebel when reporting on the case. Then, suddenly, there he was speaking to a joyous crowd in the square at the Cape Town city hall. He stepped to the balcony, a tall, gray-haired, handsome man carrying himself with the confidence of a leader who'd had a long, long time to prepare for this moment.

Two days later we sat in his garden in Soweto, the sprawling black neighborhood on the edge of Johannesburg, where he talked easily about his hopes for the future without a trace of bitterness over what he'd been through. Over the years I saw him several times in America, and I went back to South Africa in June 2013 to report on the end of his life, concentrating on the eighteen years he had spent imprisoned on Robben Island, the

stony outcrop just off Cape Town. For all its depriva-
tions, Robben Island helped shape the Nelson Mandela
we came to know later.

It is where he learned the language of the whites
from a prison guard who became his lifelong friend. In
that confined place of no physical comfort he spent
hours with his fellow political prisoners contemplating
the South Africa he'd like to lead when released, as he
was confident he would be one day.

Prison was, as it has been for so many inmates of
conscience, a harsh confinement that led him to endure
the physical pain by concentrating on that which cannot
be shackled: the mind and the liberating force of powerful ideas aligned with human rights. When word of his
death came I shared those early Mandela stories on
NBC and thought about the lessons for me in what is a
much lesser personal trial.

His life before the triumph that defined his legacy
was a reminder of the importance of patience, courage,
and the absence of self-pity. These were the same qualities that American prisoners recalled to me as the
reason they survived the brutal treatment and depriva-
tions of Japanese prisoner-of-war camps during World
War II.

Louis Zamperini, the subject of Laura Hillenbrand's
phenomenal bestseller *Unbroken*, looked surprised

when I asked if he had ever been tempted to give up while he was being tortured.

"Never," he said, adding that it was this attitude that had kept him alive.

When I met Mandela at his home in Soweto two days after his release, he might as well have been a successful businessman just returning from a trip to Zurich. The last fourteen months of his imprisonment had been spent in a South African version of a white-collar crime camp. In any case, he bore no obvious emotional scars of Robben Island or two intervening prisons. He joked with the camera crew, signed his autobiography for the children of an NBC producer, and in his answers talked of the future, not of the cruelties of the past.

A photo of me interviewing Mandela in the garden at that time is a personal treasure, all the more so now.

As the end of 2013 approached I began to read more closely accounts of the people who had died during the year, not because I was ready to check out myself but because in many instances they called up memorable relationships, occasions, or the work they left behind.

It was another reminder of the good life I've had, spending time with just a few of those who passed on: the writers Elmore Leonard and Tom Clancy; astronaut Scott Carpenter; Gene Patterson, a legendary newspaper editor; White House correspondent Helen Thomas; three Hall of Fame political journalists: Jack Germond, Anthony Lewis, and Richard Ben Cramer; Al Neuharth, fellow South Dakotan and founder of *USA Today;* former British prime minister Margaret Thatcher; pro football's Deacon Jones; Lindy Boggs, Louisiana congresswoman and mother of our friend Cokie Roberts; former Pennsylvania governor Bill Scranton, one of the last of the moderate northeastern Republicans; jazz guitarist Jim Hall.

By December it had been four months since my diagnosis and I was optimistic the treatment was going well but also apprehensive. What if my confidence was just a hangover from a life in which, despite mistakes and my imperfections, I somehow almost always emerged upright?

I'd awake nights and for just a beat forget that I had cancer. Then, the realization, the frustration, the small tick of fear that this would not end well. It was a faint fear, but I knew of too many cancer cases that seemed to be on the mend only to turn with a vengeance on the patient.

Multiple myeloma may be a small-population cancer, representing only 1 percent of the cancers recorded and affecting twenty thousand people a year, but Meredith and I keep encountering others who have the disease or who are related to myeloma patients.

One is Frank Lalli, a Sunday softball–playing buddy and former editor of *Money* magazine for Time Inc. In December 2012, eight months before my diagnosis, I was surprised to read in *The New York Times* that he had multiple myeloma. We hadn't seen each other in a while and apparently he was determined to keep his condition a private affair.

However, as an enterprising journalist who specializes in financial matters, he went public in an opinion piece that meticulously tracked his frustrations in trying to determine who would provide Revlimid when Time Warner removed the thousand-dollar cap on prescription costs for active and retired personnel alike. That meant the company would not automatically assume costs once a senior employee had spent a thousand dollars on prescriptions.

Frank quickly found himself in a wilderness of conflicting guidance and wide spreads in the cost of Revlimid, his primary chemo and maintenance drug. In one month he made seventy phone calls to sixteen organizations, including his employer, Time Warner, and Medicare. Revlimid, which has been so effective in treating myeloma, was very expensive at retail—$132,000 a year, or roughly $524 a pill.

He was stunned when he discovered that Time Warner had been spending $8,000 a month for his Revlimid. Now Time Warner was saying, in effect, "We've changed the rules. No more cap on your share of the cost. You figure it out." He was on the phone constantly to Time's health benefits officers, Medicare reps, the drug company, and the insurer. They quoted prices ranging from $20 a month to $17,000 a year.

His life was quickly divided between managing his health and managing his disputatious relationship with Time Warner on promises made and promises broken to longtime senior employees. Finally, Time Warner's insurance carrier realized that Frank was part of a subgroup that caps any specialty drug at $60 a month. He received a commitment in writing and so far it is holding up.

When I returned to New York from Minnesota I called Frank to share news of our common condition and he immediately became my pathfinder, one of those heroic World War II airborne troops who jumped in early on D-Day to guide other paratroopers to landing sites and German targets. He shared his Dana-Farber physician, Dr. Ken Anderson, as a second-opinion resource and described the various effects of drugs during the initial rounds of treatment, the criteria for choosing between stem cell transplant and drugs alone, and, most encouraging, his physical regimen, which he hoped would have him back in the batter's cage by April.

Frank was also the first but not the last to tip me to a

singular advocate for multiple myeloma patients. Kathy Giusti was diagnosed with MM in 1998 while an executive at a pharmaceutical company. She did have a successful stem cell transplant but that was before the welcome arrival of Revlimid and so her prognosis was not encouraging.

Kathy and her twin sister, Karen Andrews, a corporate attorney, decided a more businesslike approach was needed to slow this tenacious disease, so they organized MMRF, the Multiple Myeloma Research Foundation, as a central gathering place for patients, physicians, and researchers. Until Kathy and Karen got involved, a great deal of the multiple myeloma treatment and research around the world was the work of individual teams that were failing to communicate with others working on the disease. Alas, that is not an uncommon condition even in this wired world.

MMRF became, in a way, the home office of what might be called MM Inc.: that is, a foundation with a corporate attitude about making change happen quickly through innovation and an uncompromising bottom line. Is a particular treatment working? No? Move on.

As word of my condition began to seep out, I discovered that Kathy and I shared a number of friends, all uniformly enthusiastic about her personality and work. One meeting with her and I was also a member of the

Kathy Giusti admiration society. She was tuned in to all the latest developments in part because her foundation has become a central repository for work done on myeloma around the world. She has been so successful in establishing the foundation and making it a go-to resource for MM research and treatment around the world that her alma mater, Harvard Business School, has published a case study on the foundation's history and continuing influence.

My mobility and balance were steadily improving, thanks to the approach of Sloan's physical therapists. When I told them I wanted to get back to shooting and fishing they created a series of exercises to train the right muscles. We had an approximation of an uneven field in the house gym, a series of spongy pads and stools to step over or onto, gates to slide through sideways, and even a steel tube as a mock shotgun. The therapists would call out "Shoot!" as I made my way through the obstacle course, and I would turn and knock an imaginary bobwhite quail from the sky.

I seemed to do well, which helped my self-esteem, until one day when I left the gym and walked up Lexington Avenue and my hearing aid battery began to fail. It was cold and windy so I tucked up against a falafel stand and tried to change the battery with numb fingers. Fumbling, I laughed aloud at myself. "Here you are, Brokaw, sick with cancer, trying to learn to walk again, bedeviled by a hearing aid battery, and not even the falafel vendor cares. You're really pathetic."

The hearing aid is another reminder of advancing age. Hearing loss runs in the family and it is also an occupational hazard of longtime broadcasters who have had all manner of high-decibel sounds pumped into their eardrums while on the air. When Mark Leibovich wrote his withering bestseller, *This Town*, about the cultural customs and tribes of Washington, D.C., he was generous, assigning me senior status and even some wisdom. To underscore the senior status he noted I wore a hearing aid.

I wrote to say, "It's not a hearing aid; it's a Viagra drip." He asked to note that in a new edition.

Why not?

I altered other routines on the streets of New York. With my diminished strength and fragile spine I quickly discovered that Manhattan building doors require a full-body commitment to open on a cold day, of which we were having many. I'd look for someone coming through a revolving door or exiting a single-panel door and poach a ride. On subways I occasionally took the senior or handicapped seating with no hesitation or loss of pride.

My expression conveyed to fellow riders, "I'm old, dammit, sick, dammit, and get out of my face."

Well, maybe not that expression, but I was thinking it.

I missed my old life of jumping on a plane and racing off to a big breaking story. Colleagues began to remind me that the twenty-fifth anniversary of the fall of the Berlin wall was coming in November 2014, and shouldn't I be going back?

That had been a signature moment for NBC News and for me. In November 1989, our enterprising foreign editor, Jerry Lamprecht, said, "There's not much going on here; why don't you go today? East Germany is in chaos and that's a good story." I agreed and left on an overnight flight.

Our first day in the divided city was notable for the ease with which we passed through Checkpoint Charlie and into the eastern sector, where I was able to interview dissidents who spoke of the feeble attempts by the GDR—the Communist leadership of the German Democratic Republic, as they called their Moscow satellite—to deal with the restlessness of the East German citizens, hostages in their own motherland.

We had satellite capability on standby but the story, instructive and interesting, didn't measure up to the expense of a live feed, so I pretaped my segments and prepared for a second day, November 9, 1989.

Late that afternoon a GDR "information" officer, Günter Schabowski, was conducting a tendentious news conference when he inadvertently changed the course of history by mistakenly announcing new, liberal travel laws that could begin immediately. It came at the end of his news conference and as he left the room there was head-shaking confusion among the reporters. "Does this mean the wall is effectively coming down? GDR citizens can come and go as they please?"

My colleague Michele Neubert had prearranged an interview with Schabowski and so I rushed upstairs to get clarification.

Schabowski was relaxed and unapologetic about the confusion. "We have decided today to implement a regulation that allows every citizen of the German Democratic Republic to leave the GDR through any of the border crossings."

Any? I asked.

Smiling, he answered, "It is possible for them to go through the border."

We later learned that the GDR Politburo planned many stipulations for the new travel and, incredibly, thought East Germans would travel to the West and then happily return to their old lives in the East.

I ran downstairs and yelled at some American reporters puzzling over their press conference notes, "It's down, the wall. Schabowski just confirmed East Germans can exit through any border crossing."

By the time we got to Checkpoint Charlie the word was out on the streets of East Germany and the GDR guard didn't bother looking through our car when we stopped for inspection. I asked what he thought of the news. He offered a small smile and said, "I am not paid to think."

At other crossing points, notably the Bornholmer Strasse bridge and checkpoint, GDR guards were attempting to deal with the rapid buildup of East Germans who wanted to go through the wall. They were getting little or no guidance from their superiors. The guards briefly wondered whether they were expected to shoot the demonstrators.

At Rockefeller Center in New York my colleague Garrick Utley, a longtime student of German history and politics, got in the anchor chair and interviewed me on my car phone. Others made sure the satellite booking was still good, and I raced to our office to prepare for that evening.

We began to get reports of crowds of West German students congregating on their side of the wall at the Brandenburg Gate, which was also our satellite transmission site. By the time I arrived it was like a pep rally, with the western students shouting at the young on the eastern side, in effect, "Come on over!"

GDR guards unleashed their water hoses, driving the students from the wall for a short time, but when the water stopped, the students returned, resuming their recruiting cries to the young in the East. We were very close to broadcast time and still we didn't have video of East Germans actually crossing.

Then one of our cameramen arrived from the Bornholmer Strasse bridge, breathless, with the video we needed. The guards had decided not to shoot and, getting no coherent direction from their superiors, had opened the bridge to the West. The wall was breached.

At the Brandenburg Gate the water hoses trickled down as the West German students refused to leave, keeping up their shouted encouragement to those gathered on the eastern side. Then, suddenly, a young East German popped atop the wall, cheered by his generational new friends from the West, looking at once startled, apprehensive, and then happy when he was not hauled down by GDR guards.

At NBC News we had a worldwide television exclusive and I thought, "My god, this video will be around forever." So I discarded the backcountry jacket I'd brought to Germany and relieved my colleague Mike Boettcher of a handsome blue topcoat he'd just bought in London.

It was so noisy and generally chaotic that just before

we went on the air I told Bill Wheatley, the executive producer, and our control room producer, Cheryl Gould, in New York, "Just stay with me. I'm going to have to ad-lib most of this." We opened with the unexpected scenes of throngs of East Germans on foot and in their tiny Lada automobiles, pouring through the wall at several checkpoints. It was a television moment that twinned the historic if confusing policy change with the visual effect of the announcement.

I stayed on the air after *Nightly* for updates and a late evening special report in which I asked for an opportunity to reflect on the changes I had witnessed as a journalist in my twenty-seven years on the job.

For me, 1968 had always been the year in bold print, when Lyndon Johnson was forced to step aside as president because his Vietnam policies caused such a revolt in the Democratic Party that he was in danger of losing the nomination to Senator Eugene McCarthy of Minnesota. Then Senator Robert F. Kennedy entered the race and was assassinated just after midnight on the day following his victory in the California primary.

Earlier, Dr. Martin Luther King, Jr., was murdered in Memphis as he prepared for a rally on behalf of striking sanitation workers. Sixteen thousand American military men were dying in Vietnam. The Democratic National Convention in Chicago was riotous inside and outside the hall. The racist governor of Alabama, George C. Wallace, declared for president, joining Hubert Humphrey for the Democrats and Richard M. Nixon for the Republicans in the contest. At the end of the year the astronauts of *Apollo* 8 became the first men to orbit the moon.

Standing at the Brandenburg Gate, I reminded our audience of 1968, saying I had never expected to experience such a newsworthy year again. However, in 1989 a new world was being formed. With Mikhail Gorbachev as the reform-minded general secretary of the Soviet Communist Party, the most powerful position in Russia, the Soviet satellites were moving toward independence. I was in Prague the night the Velvet Revolution separated Czechoslovakia from Moscow's rule and spent time in Poland with the charismatic Lech Walesa, who led Solidarity.

Nineteen eighty-nine was that kind of year. Earlier, in June, I finished a commencement address at Tulane University School of Medicine on a Saturday morning and got a call from our news desk: Chinese troops had moved on young urban protesters who had taken over Tiananmen Square in the heart of the Chinese capital, demanding more political and personal freedom after a state visit from Gorbachev, who was reforming Soviet political oppression.

By Sunday, June 4, we knew that many of the demonstrators had been killed by the army troops trucked into

Beijing from the countryside. The capital was effectively under military rule.

I decided to go. It wasn't easy. In Tokyo a helpful Pan Am agent explained that commercial flights were out of the question but that some governments were flying in supplies to their embassies. I made a middle-of-the-night appeal to Secretary of State James Baker to let me on an American supply flight. His aide called back. "Sorry. No."

My new friend from Pan Am pulled some strings and I hopped aboard a British charter filled with food and medical supplies for the United Kingdom embassy.

Arriving in Beijing was an eerie experience. One of the world's largest and most energetic cities was as quiet as a small town in Iowa on a summer day. Military guards were at every intersection and the normal, very heavy bicycle traffic was greatly reduced. For the first two days we relied on material from state television and what little we could record on backstreets in Beijing to describe the crackdown and the shake-up of the Chinese government, orchestrated by the diminutive but tough Deng Xiaoping. Deng knew that to survive China had to reform economically but he insisted the changes had to come from the top down, not from the streets.

On the third day one of my favorite cameramen, Tony Wasserman, who had flown in from South Africa, was fiddling with a cardboard box on the back rack of a Flying Pigeon bicycle, the ubiquitous form of transportation used by the average Chinese.

"What's up?" I asked. My bearded friend in his African bush shorts grinned, held up a small video camera, and said, "Mate, I think we can make some pictures."

We secreted the camera in the box with a small hole for the lens and took off for Tiananmen, me following behind on my own Flying Pigeon, which, as I remember, we got for twenty bucks from a used Flying Pigeon lot.

It worked. We rode past parked tanks in the square, armed guards everywhere and Mao's outsize portrait on display as I described the scenes and the new climate of fear and military omnipresence. Just one Chinese cyclist caught on, pedaling up to the back of Tony's bike and tickling the lens through the peephole.

We expanded our territory to some of the backstreets and markets on our second day, prompting a memorable encounter. A student rode up to my parked bike, looked around cautiously, and whispered, "Changing China—we need more and more of the Voice of America."

He was referring to a weeklong series of reports NBC News broadcast from throughout China in 1985, as the pace of change was picking up under the direction of Deng. Beijing was becoming a modern capital, with luxurious hotels and free-enterprise cafés. The hutongs, rudimentary communal villages in the heart of Beijing, were being cleared to make way for high-rise apartments and stores carrying Ralph Lauren, Nike, and other high-profile Western goods.

I wanted to visit Tibet, I said to Beijing officials, the Buddhist kingdom now under the military if not the spiritual control of the Chinese government. Han Chinese who had no appreciation of the Tibetan culture were being shipped in from the country's coastal areas to take up residence and the government infrastructure was under the control of Beijing. The Chinese government was happy to help until they discovered that my carefully arranged five-day trip to Tibet was not a feature on tourism. I was determined to show how the Beijing rulers were systematically trying to wipe out any memory of His Holiness the Dalai Lama, who had fled to India with the help of the American CIA in 1959.

Meredith and I flew to Lhasa, the exotic capital, elevation just short of twelve thousand feet, and took in the monumental Potala Palace, where we shared a cup of rancorous yak butter tea, the local specialty, with a picnicking Tibetan family. It was a cordial and useful ceremony, for we learned how hospitable the Tibetan people would be and how to forevermore feign an appreciation for yak butter tea.

Chinese officials rolled out the Panchen Lama, the second-ranking lama, who stayed behind when His Holiness fled to India, becoming Beijing's front man in the government's attempt to say all is well in the Holy Land.

He was a large man of few words who carried himself with the physical weariness of an actor in a role he reluctantly filled. With Han Chinese officials monitoring our conversation, he invited us to his home temple, Tashilhunpo Monastery in Xigazê, a sprawling city southwest of Lhasa reached by a tortuous mountain road under constant repair by work gangs with shovels and, when we were there, no heavy construction equipment.

Our guesthouse quarters were just above pigsty standards. Fortunately we had our own sleeping bags, some water, and food from Lhasa. When I walked into our room Meredith said quickly, "Don't touch a thing."

I said, "I thought no hot water."

She said, "Right."

I pointed to an exposed lighting fixture in the ceiling in which water was pouring down a bare electrical wire, hitting the cement floor boiling hot.

At dawn the next morning we were escorted into an ancient chanting room at the monastery, which dates to the fifteenth century. It was a mystical scene, lit by yak butter lamps and the first rays of a new day making their way through cracked and dirty windows at the back. The ocher-colored wooden pillars had a dusky hue, exposed as they have been to centuries of smoke from candles and heaters fueled by yak dung.

Rows of wooden benches in a kind of amphitheater

were filled with pubescent boys and their elders ranging in age from late teens to what appeared to be many in their eighties or nineties. All were wrapped in crimson robes trimmed in gold as they answered the head priest who led the chanting, pausing occasionally for a yak butter tea break. The tea was served by strong-armed teenagers who walked through the congregation with four-foot-long ornate wooden pitchers, replenishing the small wooden bowls that had been tucked into the robes of the faithful.

Meredith sat quietly at the back, surely one of the few Anglo women ever to attend morning services. We were both deeply impressed by the devotion to their faith of the priests, a faith that had no discernible connection to the central government in Beijing.

When we returned to Lhasa I decided to test the insistence of our Chinese minders that the self-exiled Dalai Lama no longer had any standing in Tibet. We sent our minder on a "shopping trip" with Meredith while producer Charlie Ryan and cameraman Gary Fairman and I began a casual walk counterclockwise around Jokhang Temple, the most sacred place in Tibet. Buddhist pilgrims, many on their hands and knees, come from afar to circle the temple clockwise, hands clasped, eyes cast downward. These devotionals have been going on since the temple was built in 647, the beginning of Tibetan Buddhism.

As a pilgrim approached I withdrew a postcard of the Dalai Lama I had smuggled into Tibet and held it at eye level. The reaction was instant and emotional. One after another, pilgrims reached out for the image, many of them moaning and weeping.

So much for the claim that the Dalai Lama had no standing.

Our minder returned and went ballistic, demanding the video we had shot. We gave him a blank roll of tape and agreed to leave the next day. Back in Beijing, our official hosts, senior government officers, were even more exercised, abandoning their English language skills and speaking to us only through interpreters, threatening to shut down the weeklong project and throw us out. The dispute was still unresolved when Meredith and I, celebrating our twenty-fifth wedding anniversary, flew off to Dharamsala, the northern Indian home in exile of the Dalai Lama, to share with His Holiness what we had recorded.

We were guests in what amounts to a small, well-organized city in the foothills of the Himalayas, the center of the exiled government. We found ourselves unprepared for our host's robust personality and utter absence of aloofness. Here was a man considered by his followers to be a living god and yet he had the demeanor of a successful mayor, a hearty handshake and boisterous laugh. He quieted when we loaded the videotape for screening and watched intently scenes shot in places he had not seen for decades. When the Panchen Lama appeared on the screen he inquired about his health but said nothing about his relationship with the Beijing government.

In 1989, when the Panchen Lama died of a heart attack at the age of fifty-one, stories began to leak out that he was a behind-the-scenes critic of Beijing's crackdown on Buddhism and that, following the Cultural Revolution, he had argued for the restoration of the Tibetan language as the official language of the region. He had also publicly proclaimed his personal and spiritual friendship with the Dalai Lama.

In Dharamsala we were invited to witness His Holiness at morning prayer in a corner of his modest home, which resembled a fifties ranch-style house on the outer reaches of Malibu. First, he listened to the world news from the BBC on a portable radio, and then, sitting lotus-style, he launched into the prayers. I understood not a word, but the muscular recitation that went on for half an hour was irresistible. When I told him how moved I had been he laughed, grabbed my hand, and gave me the living god's version of a fist bump.

I flew back to Beijing with a worldwide exclusive: the first network interview with the Dalai Lama, accompanied by supporting video from inside Tibet. By now the Chinese government was apoplectic. I asked Winston Lord, the U.S. ambassador to China, if there was any way to broadcast my reporting and not get thrown out. He was pessimistic, saying Chinese officials might ban NBC from doing any business in China.

Just then, a bulletin on the newswires: Lamas in Lhasa were rioting in protest of Chinese suppression of their beliefs, and the Han Chinese military had been called in to suppress the protest. I had a lead for my reporting and the Chinese officials let the transmission go out.

In the years since, I've seen His Holiness several times and I keep within view of my NBC desk a portrait of the two of us, laughing, as he drapes a prayer shawl over my shoulders.

Meredith keeps in a safe a ring he gave her as a gesture of friendship, not engagement, I presume.

Those are the experiences I don't want to confine to memory. I understand I'll be in a slower lane even if I put this cancer behind me but I do not want to become a Tommy-sit-by-the-fire. As for the treatment, by the first week of December we'd know the results from the late round of Revlimid as measured by the blood samples, the PET scan, and the bone marrow extraction. It had been four full months since my diagnosis and I was living the new normal.

Normal now meant the daily drugs, the on-again, off-again back pains, the fatigue, and the uncertain walking gait. I wanted to shed the new normal and get back to the old model. These results would be a barometer of whether that was possible.

There was no reason to believe the worst. My first tests had been so positive. Apart from the episodic, piercing back pain I was highly mobile and sleeping through the night, interrupted only by a soaking of night sweats in my upper right torso. The sweats were a nuisance and a little mysterious. They arrived in a burst about 2:00 A.M., soaked my T-shirt, and then shut down. What triggered them? They are not unusual in cancer cases and the exact cause remains uncertain, but given the diet of drugs and physiological changes in a cancer patient's body the choices were many.

Nocturnal sweating was a minor concern as we made our way through the Sloan Kettering corridors. I was a little apprehensive. What if the earlier progress had stalled or other trouble signs had developed?

Dr. Landau arrived and in her steady, businesslike fashion got immediately to the point. It was all good news. There had been a 90 percent drop in M protein, one of the key indicators. Plasma cells, the central villain when they become cancerous, went from 60 percent affected to 5 to 10 percent. The PET scan showed bone quality just below normal. Dr. Landau finished the report card and said to me, "We don't need to do a stem cell transplant. We can continue with drugs but we'll harvest stem cells just in case. That begins next week."

Her judgment is a vivid example of how rapidly treatment for multiple myeloma is changing. A year ago, with the same results, she might have chosen a transplant as the next step.

Now I had to hope standby stem cells could be harvested without too much difficulty. My aging veins wouldn't support a venal hookup to the blood collection machinery so they drilled a small hole in my upper right torso and inserted a two-way catheter with colored caps—one for outgoing blood, the other for a return once the stem cells had been separated.

The catheter had the appearance of primitive jewelry or perhaps an award to a Masai warrior for bravery in the field. I felt neither brave nor bejeweled. I simply wanted to get on with it, four days prone on a hospital bed, giving and receiving a steady stream from the five liters of blood most of us have coursing through our system, red and white cells each with a specific assignment.

The weekend before the procedure began I injected myself with two drugs designed to loosen the stem cell platelets, the baby blood cells, and store them separately. Repeat the do-it-yourself injection the morning of the first procedure and take another drug orally. A breakfast heavy in calcium is recommended to ward off chills. Veterans of the procedure called to say, "Take lots of books and other reading material. There's nothing else to do while you're there."

Not for the first time during various treatments and office waits for results, I was very grateful for the digital tablet. Seldom do I have four uninterrupted hours for newspapers, email, books, or online shopping. The downside? The drugs, especially a powerful one at the end of the day, leave you vaguely unsettled physically, one more reminder of the pervasive forces of the disease and the efforts to control it. The out-of-sight fight between drugs and rogue cells for dominance in your bloodstream can be exhausting physically and emotionally.

The drive to and from Sloan in the evening dusk showed off the city in its holiday dress. The red, silver, and green glow from decorated Christmas trees framed by apartment windows and elaborately lit entrances to town houses were welcome distractions from the clinical settings of my destination and reminders of better days.

Four consecutive mornings I checked in at the blood donor offices and took my place in a curtained-off bed at the end of a ward where cheerful Jane, a nurse originally from Puerto Rico, hooked me up to a blood machine designed to draw off stem cells, those newbies that have not yet decided whether to be oxygen-generating red cells or disease-fighting white blood cells. Four hours later I was on my way home and by midafternoon Dr. Reichel, the Argentine American, called to report that the harvest had been modestly successful and that she would see me tomorrow.

Three more sessions were required and by Friday noon I was en route to a welcome distraction: A French producer had enlisted me to narrate an IMAX 3-D all-digital depiction of D-Day, seventy years ago, June 6, 1944.

When first approached I was reluctant because there have been so many D-Day productions, including three that I've reported on for NBC News. However, a preview of the French enterprise quickly won me over. The digital re-creation frees the producers from the same old grainy black-and-white film and allows them to put on the screen with heretofore unseen clarity the big picture and the smallest detail. For the first time, viewers can see the invasion armada from starboard to port, bow to stern. The Norman shoreline and countryside are faithfully reproduced, from Cherbourg to Caen, with the various German units, their size and mission, rising out of the digital landscape. Stylish portraits of General Dwight D. Eisenhower and the other principal commanders emerge from the screen at the appropriate moments.

To have a part in this enterprise, which was being produced for young people and to be shown in museums in the West, allowed me again to keep my condition in perspective. I wasn't getting off a landing craft in heavy surf at dawn to face murderous fire with the odds short that I would survive fifteen minutes.

The narration went well, with the exception of my inability to nail the final nuanced syllable of "Bayeux," the charming Norman city where I usually stay when I am in that part of the world. Finally, I got it right, or so the crew assured me. With a departing gift of vintage Calvados I was on my way to a family reunion for the holidays, thinking the tough December path was at an end.

Wrong again.

Walking into our home in the woods north of the city two days before Christmas I had my arms full of packages and in the dark failed to see a newly formed ledge leading to a flagstone patio. Suddenly I was falling, hard, face-first onto the patio. I was furious and frightened. I could feel the first steady stream of blood from somewhere. My glasses were smashed. Oddly, my head didn't hurt as much as it seemed it should. I sat up slowly, bleeding down my jacket, grateful I had not been knocked out. My eyesight seemed intact.

My body was bruised but not broken. I made it into the house and called for Meredith to meet me in the bathroom. My face was a mess. A deep, jagged wound was open over my left eye and there were other contusions.

Meredith rushed me to a nearby emergency room—"Tom Brokaw, two six four oh"—where the staff ran some basic tests to determine if my vision and cognitive skills had been affected. Luckily, a plastic surgeon was on call and stitched me up so precisely—three layers deep—that three months later there was not a trace of an opening that went right to the skull bone.

By 10:00 we were back home and I fixed Meredith a stiff martini, grateful again she was at my side. Over the years she's seen me through a serious helicopter crash, a deadly river-running trip, broken ankles, feet, and fingers, assorted parasitic conditions from the Middle East, and an anthrax attack on my office. Now cancer and a flagstone face-plant.

Her reaction is always the same: "We'll get through this. A year from now will be much better." One of her friends used to comment on Meredith's steely resolve masked by her ethereal beauty. Over the years I've come to take it for granted, that combination of compassion and cool determination. She's been a board member for Gannett, the media conglomerate, and for nonprofits such as Channel 13 and Conservation International. I'd get these glowing reports from others about her low-key but invaluable contributions on initiatives and her quiet refusal to be rolled on dubious proposals from management.

When I'd share that feedback with her she'd shrug it off. I'm the bombastic branch of the family. She's the modest, still-water-runs-deep branch.

During my illness I kept waiting for her to suggest nothing more daring than a Barcalounger, but then she's taken our daughters on a glacier trek in the Hunza Valley of northern Pakistan, our granddaughters to the Galápagos and on whale-watching excursions, and ridden horseback with girlfriends into the Montana wilderness. She's so attached to these horse outings she joined an Icelandic horse safari across a long stretch of that North Atlantic country and also rode into the remote reaches of Patagonia. She completed the New York City Marathon in four hours while running her small chain of toy stores.

Three other friends dealing with debilitating health issues volunteer that their wives are performing the same heroics in much the same fashion. We three generally wind up conversations with a rare show of humility, acknowledging how lucky we are to have married such strong, capable, and uncomplaining women. "Awe" is not too strong as a description of our reaction.

What's left unspoken is this: Would I be as helpful

and generous if the roles were reversed? God, I hope so, but I also recognize that Meredith, as an expert bridge player, Scrabble fanatic, hostess, cook, benefit organizer, and businesswoman, is happiest when the job at hand requires a finely tuned detail gene.

That is never more evident than during the Christmas holidays, when, as we like to say in our family, it's all about Baby Jesus and Meredith.

December 25 is her birthday as well and despite the conventional reaction—"Oh, dear, too bad; you must get short-changed"—the holiday is especially rich in our family as we celebrate Christ's birthday and Meredith in all of her glory.

She spends weeks planning and preparing the Christmas Eve guest list and menu: country ham and homemade biscuits; oyster stew; fresh oysters and clams; endive filled with crab salad; game sausages from Montana; Christmas pudding from her own recipe; old-fashioned Christmas cookies and magnums of Champagne followed by Christmas caroling.

Every year, the same promise: "This is my last year. I can't do all this work every year." Yet, with the exception of her sixty-fifth birthday, which we celebrated in Hawaii, she's back at it shortly after Thanksgiving.

The arrival of the first grandson, Sarah's Archer, gave the occasion an extra glow. His girl cousins inducted him into the Christmas-morning ritual of opening presents and posing for pictures taken by the ubiquitous cell phone cameras.

I raised a glass to Meredith and all that she and the family mean to me in the best of circumstances, a compact that has been tested and strengthened during this cancer blindside. To keep from choking up I invoked some locker-room language to bid farewell to 2013, saying the New Year was welcome and bound to be better.

It did have a promising beginning. I was largely pain-free and the decision not to undergo a stem cell transplant meant we could plan some time out of the city in the coming months, joining friends in the Caribbean, visiting Sarah and Archer in Los Angeles. I'd already given up six months of my old life, and, unrealistically, I kept thinking I could reclaim it just around the next treatment.

In February I turned seventy-four with none of the old panache: "Bring it on—trips to war zones and bike trips in Chile. Fishing in the Bahamas and maybe a week in China." For the first time I began to acknowledge limits and concentrated on a different kind of calendar: Will I be there when the youngest granddaughters, Vivian and Charlotte Bird, head off to college? How will being a single mom to Archer work out for Sarah in the long haul? The San Francisco branch, Claire and Meredith, so gifted and promising, let me see their full realization.

Selectively I reentered the public arena, interviewing my old friend Jane Pauley on her new book about the choices baby boomers can make for the back third of their lives. We first met when she was the *Today Show* ingénue in the midseventies. Now here she is, a kind of youthful grande dame of boomers, still slyly witty.

Jane told the audience, "Baby boomers are often misunderstood. We didn't invent sex, drugs, and rock and roll, but we took it to scale."

My schedule was carefully calibrated so I could be home by 8:00 P.M. or so. Some evenings were harder to leave than others.

The National Board of Review is a New York organization of film critics, academicians, publicists, and others in the entertainment business who know how to attract attention: put on an award show leading up to the Academy Awards. This year my longtime friend George Stevens, Jr., son of the late legendary director, was being honored for establishing the American Film Institute, producing and directing his own films, and presiding over the Kennedy Center Honors. I was privileged to pay tribute to George but I knew I'd have to leave shortly after. It was not easy. The room was in a giddy mood, with Meryl Streep and Emma Thompson lighting up the festivities with wicked takes on Walt Disney and women in high heels.

Bruce Dern stopped by to ask Meredith if she was still running marathons. Leonardo DiCaprio and Martin Scorsese did a comic riff. Steve McQueen, the director of *12 Years a Slave,* was honored and gave a heartfelt speech.

Or so I read the next day. I was home in bed by 8:45, a long way from my early days in New York, when Jane Pauley would joke I stayed out half the night because I was afraid of the dark.

Just as I was beginning to plot a return to almost normal, during the summer months back pain made a return visit. Persistent and more aggravating than debilitating, it again became a constant companion, a reminder that maybe my track to recovery had more detours than I had expected.

An MRI was scheduled while I was negotiating an interview with Greg Mortenson, his first since *60 Minutes* raised serious questions about his phenomenal bestseller, *Three Cups of Tea,* an inspirational account of building schools for girls in Afghanistan. There were also allegations of financial abuses and exaggerated claims of success. Mortenson was forced to resign from his foundation, pay back a million dollars, and rethink his life.

Since I knew Greg, his family, his work, and his accusers, I was in a unique position to conduct the first interview with him since the scandal broke. I warned him and his friends it would not be softball. It was not, and he rose to the occasion, admitting that he made mistakes, that he apologized to staff members who early on raised flags about the abuses. He also thanked Steve Kroft of *60 Minutes* and author-mountaineer Jon Krakauer, who first raised the issues, saying they probably saved his life because he was forced to concentrate on his health, including a serious cardiac condition.

Greg, the son of Lutheran missionaries, was the classic victim of that ancient Greek disease hubris. He now recognizes that and wants only to return to building schools and educating young Afghan women, leaving the foundation and fund-raising in the hands of others. He was grateful for the direct questions and the opportunity to begin anew. I reminded him America is a land of redemption if you admit your mistakes. He is a young man with a big heart and a determination to change the lives of young women in one of the most gender-hostile places on earth, northern Afghanistan. He's now back at it.

Once the Mortenson interview was out of the way I appeared for my MRI, which lasted about an hour. I had no sense of foreboding, which was a routine Brokaw approach. "Everything will be just fine."

Wrong.

I had several compression factures along my spine, including an ugly one at a location called T12, in the midback area. Strung together, they were like an alarm system, but what were they signaling? Had the myeloma flared up? Were my bones more fragile than we thought? Did I imprudently lift objects that were too heavy?

Most important, why hadn't the physician in charge of my physical rehabilitation picked up on the developing fractures earlier? Perhaps my threshold for pain was misleading. When I said my pain level was a two-three on a scale of ten, would others have identified the same pain as a five-six?

On every visit from September through December I acknowledged pain, but never at an acute level. Nonetheless, its persistence should have prompted a hands-on physical run down my spine to determine if there were sensitive areas. That did not happen, for whatever reason.

The Sloan specialist in charge of structural issues was a forty-three-year-old with a big résumé, a brusque style, and apparently not much interest in face-to-face consultation, for I saw him only twice from September to January. He was another reminder of the importance of becoming proactive in your treatment.

At the same time I was losing height. Through my

fifties I was an even six feet and then dropped down to five eleven. Now I was aware of standing next to old friends and feeling much shorter than in earlier encounters. In fact, I was. I measured five feet nine, just barely. That was alarming. Was I becoming a man shrunken by disease and an unstable spine? Good god, what next?

What next was a procedure called kyphoplasty, in which the patient is under general anesthesia while neurosurgeons or specially trained radiologists shore up the fractures with cement injected through a needle. I felt like a pothole on the highway of life.

There was some discussion of bracing the T12 fracture with a rod and screws but in a quick survey of other specialists arranged by Jennifer, the consensus was "stay away from that kind of invasion."

In the pre-op discussion I was startled to hear the radiologist say that if they had detected these fractures in November, say, he could have cemented them in their infancy, which would have been preferable.

I had grown up with a father for whom pain was a personal burden, not to be shared with others. During his severe back injuries he'd come home at the end of a long workday, strip off his shirt, make some iced tea, and sit in a straight-back chair, staring blankly at the far wall, never whining. I was never that stoic but I did inherit some of his attitude.

Two memories: I severely wrenched my left ankle when it was caught on a sagebrush stem as we rushed by in an ATV during Montana hunting season. On the advice of a hunting companion, a brother-in-law who is an ob-gyn, I iced it that night, laced up my boot extra-tight the next day, and hunted again. By the day after that the swelling was alarming and Dr. Jennifer insisted I go to the emergency room, which I did, reluctantly. X rays showed I had snapped my distal left fibula, the slender bone leading to the heel.

As Jennifer tartly reminded me, if I were going to have a baby, listen to the beloved ob-gyn brother-in-law, but severe ankle pain required a different kind of attention.

In our physician-intense clan, that is now part of the family lore.

The other memory is of a ring finger jammed during a Sunday softball game. It hurt but I thought I could play on, especially after two teammates, one a veterinarian and the other a psychiatrist, examined it and tried to pop it back in place. After the game, in rural Connecticut, a local physician looked at it and said, "Get to the Hospital for Special Surgery in New York right away. It is all but destroyed." And so it was. After a long microsurgery and an overnight stay in the hospital I had a new, much more expensive finger, with or without a ring.

The veterinarian and the psychiatrist decided not to open a digital repair practice.

"Tom Brokaw, two six four oh." On the morning of the kyphoplasty I had another of my Sloan immigrant nation moments. An attendant in the operating theater had a distinctive accent and so I asked about her origins. "Russia," she said, smiling. "I lived all over Russia, went to medical school there, and then came here and went to medical school again." With that I went under, awakening two hours later to the radiologist reporting it had all gone well. He was pleased he had managed to make repairs on that ugly T12 fracture.

I walked out under my own power and with Meredith at my side we headed for home for twenty-four hours of downtime and then a tempered physical routine.

The pain did not disappear. Three days after the kyphoplasty I was in more pain than expected, especially in the longitudinal muscles on either side of the spine. My spirits sagged and I gave in to some unexpected weeping brought on, I think, by drugs, the uncertainty of my recovery, and the absence of ANY relief from the omnipresence of cancer.

Some of the emotional spillover came from positive personal experiences, such as conversations with Jennifer in which she offered a spot-on analysis of what should be done next in my case or a touching and yet hilarious description of brother Bill's latest eruption at his assisted living facility. I'd hang up, still laughing but also weepy with pride in all that she'd become.

Her nickname among friends at medical school was "Bombs-Away Brokaw" for her take-no-prisoners style when it came to ethical issues, tough medical decisions, or personal behavior. Yet what she loved most about medicine was her ability to help people. She spent a year before medical school in the dangerous Pakistani border town of Peshawar, working with Afghan women refugees fleeing the Russian occupation of their country.

She went into the rudimentary camps, dressed in the wardrobe of a Muslim woman, and counseled women on fundamental issues of female health. Their instant response was so gratifying she decided she wanted to be a hands-on, help-right-now kind of doctor, so she began to think emergency room medicine instead of infectious diseases, which had been her first choice.

Jennifer's assistance in my case was one of the many unanticipated benefits. Shortly after my diagnosis I had a heightened awareness of what the diagnostic team did not tell me. During my first visit to Sloan a number of physicians and administrators stopped by to cheerily assure me I was in good hands and several said something to the effect of "You'll be back to your old form by spring."

That was reassuring but overly optimistic. Jennifer was more realistic, counseling me that my old life would have to be shelved and that I would need to concentrate full-time on being a cancer patient. Even with her warning I was not prepared for the precipitous weight loss, the effect of compression fractures in my back, and the diminished muscle tone.

Meredith, who sat in on all of the meetings, correctly thinks the projection of what lies ahead in a cancer case is a combination of physicians enlisting the patient in a best-case scenario and the patients not fully comprehending the pernicious effect of cancer on their physical, mental, and emotional makeup.

I quickly learned multiple myeloma would dictate the terms of my life, from physical fitness to summer schedules to appetite to energy to appreciation of my surroundings.

Two years ago we moved from our large, two-story apartment into a pied-à-terre, a much smaller place but all we need to nest in our neighborhood. Meredith pulled it all together in a fashion reflecting our life divided between New York and the West. Evocative western landscapes, rare Bodmer prints, and a collection of equine art showing off horses on the run and at rest, all framing elongated windows looking over Central Park and the Upper East Side.

Until MM struck I loved to sit in front of a fire in the living room, a drink in hand and a history book off the shelves, absorbed by the comfort of the surroundings. Now when I moved into that room the art, books, and fireplace became minor characters on the stage of a life dominated by the pain or anxiety of myeloma. Cancer becomes the scrim through which all of life is viewed.

I hoped that as time passed I would be able to raise the cancer shade and allow more light into my daily life. Until then it is CANCER EVERY WAKING MOMENT and the realization that it will be with me until the end, by whatever means.

It is this uncompromising reality that should motivate every cancer patient, and patients afflicted with any kind of complicated condition, to constantly ask, "Is this the right approach? Am I making the progress expected?" Most important, are all the parts of my treatment team working together? On big decisions of consequence, are they figuratively or literally at the table at the same time or on the same computer screen?

There came a moment when I decided that beginning with Dr. Landau I was in the hands of gifted individual physicians. All the same, communication between them was spotty or absent altogether at some critical moments.

Were we being sufficiently aggressive? Why weren't

all members of the team present for big decisions, either online or on the telephone or in the room? I was especially unhappy with that physician supposedly in charge of my structural issues. Following kyphoplasty he remained missing in action. Without seeing me in person he sent to a Sloan physical therapist a chart showing the devices I would need for everyday activity, including a walker, an elaborate plastic sleeve for pulling on socks, and detailed instructions on how to exit a car. I was prepared for changes in my life but this seemed over the top, and the radiologist who performed the procedure agreed. "Just use your head," he said. "Don't do anything radical and you should be fine."

He did warn me against any activity that would torque the spine, such as golf, horseback riding, shooting, or muscular fly casting. As a Jersey boy he had no appreciation of the difference between casting for a 3-pound bonefish and going to sea for a 150-pound marlin, so I sent videos of bonefishing.

I laughed when he told me he tried to duplicate the motions with a cheap spinning rod in his backyard.

What was not a laughing matter was my growing discomfort with the lack of shared dialogue in my treatment. With the exception of the MIA physical rehab physician, all the doctors were individually attentive, but rarely did I feel they were wearing the same team colors.

Immodestly, I knew I was a high-profile patient, but I was determined to have a low-profile demeanor. Through living in a family of physicians, my experience on the Mayo board, and reporting three healthcare documentaries, I knew the daily pressure on doctors. In complicated cases, it seems to me that the patient-team relationship should be seamless and all-inclusive.

By then I had established a regular telephone relationship with Dr. Ken Anderson, of Dana-Farber at Harvard, a seminal figure in developing and applying the new drug treatments working so well in MM cases. He had been Geraldine Ferraro's doctor throughout, his care no doubt helping her to live much longer than the usual MM life span at the time. He has devoted forty years of his career to what he calls "this nasty disease." From patients and experts alike, any mention of his name would elicit strong encomiums: "He's the best, and such a nice guy."

With daughter Jennifer on a conference call we reviewed my case and I asked if Ken could join the team. By then I knew he was familiar with Dr. Landau and saw her as a bright young oncologist with a growing reputation in the treatment of MM. He said he would be honored.

I was flattered but said once he got to know me he'd get over the "honored" part.

When I shared the details of our conversation with Dr. Landau she was on board immediately. Anderson wanted to go to heavier artillery, adding a drug called Velcade. As he said, "Some hospitals save Velcade for the worst-case scenario. I believe if you have myeloma, it is the worst case."

Dr. Landau worried some about a side effect, neuropathy, in which the patient gets a burning sensation in the feet or tingling in the hands. I decided I could handle some of that if it would advance the larger goal of getting MM under control. Neuropathy did show up but it was a minor case of numbness on the soles of my feet, affecting my gait some but not enough to be a distraction. It was another of the instructive passages in this journey as a patient faced with big decisions in the treatment of a life-threatening disease.

Whatever the disease, patients have to be their own advocates and, if possible, have access to a physician not on the primary team, someone who can translate medical language and ask the questions only another physician would know. This is a reality the medical profession is slowly beginning to recognize, but institutional pride and a long history of not interfering or commenting on another physician's approach is deeply rooted.

The role of the patient is equally freighted with traditional attitudes and changing expectations. Even with the advantages of a high personal profile, a family physician at my side, personal relationships with Sloan trustees, and a wide range of solicited and unsolicited opinions about whether to make changes, the decision to bring in another doctor is not just another button on speed dial. Adding Ken Anderson of Dana-Farber to the team did not go unnoticed at the highest echelons of Sloan, but no one questioned my judgment or right to make the call. I described him as my offensive coordinator, with Dr. Landau the play-calling quarterback, the physician who would move the ball down the field. I needed both and each had a critical role.

Medicine is a science but it is not physics, in which so many of the laws are certain. Medical science has its own dynamic and the human body is constantly presenting new challenges to whatever attempts are made to take control of it on our terms. Three physicians at the top of their profession may look at a complicated problem through three different prisms. Which to trust?

In dealing with the Soviet Union during the tense negotiations on reducing nuclear stockpiles, President Ronald Reagan liked to say, "Trust, but verify," a mantra he quoted so often that Soviet leader Mikhail Gorbachev finally threw up his hands and said the Russian equivalent of "Enough already."

Patients with complicated life-altering or potentially

life-ending conditions would do well to adopt the "trust, but verify" reminder.

Once my condition became more widely known a number of people urged me to confer with Dr. Jerome Groopman, the Harvard Medical School professor who is also a gifted journalist, writing in *The New Yorker* with clarity and style about health and medical matters. I resisted, saying that he was a busy man and that our shared profession of journalism didn't give me license to disrupt his life. Maureen Dowd, the *New York Times* columnist, was so persistent I thought she might have me kidnapped and delivered to him in the trunk of a car. Dr. Groopman had saved a member of her family with his treatment of a blood condition.

So I called, and my earlier resistance suddenly seemed foolish. Even over the telephone he was avuncular. He was quick to praise Dr. Anderson and the treatment course under way. We talked as well about his guidebooks for patients, *Your Medical Mind—How to Decide What Is Right for You* and *How Doctors Think.*

Together or separately they're Baedekers for patients entering the realm of modern medicine and choices, often life and death choices. In *Your Medical Mind* Groopman and his coauthor, Pamela Hartzband, MD, who also happens to be his wife, cite contemporary research on the doctor-patient relationship, but the most telling stories are case studies.

They recount the case of Julie, a smart, disciplined owner of an upscale art gallery who through self-examination and confirmation from oncologists discovered she had an aggressive form of breast cancer. She wanted the "best of the best" to treat her. A friend found the man and so she called to say, "I would really like to come in and talk to you about my situation and understand what the options are and what you recommend."

He was headed to a conference in Europe and wouldn't be able to see her for a week but that did not diminish his self-confidence. "There's really no need for a lot of discussion," he said, "I know what is best for you. You're going to get great care here." He paused before adding, "I guarantee you're going to love us."

Julie immediately thought, "I don't know that I am going to love you."

The self-assured doctor, the Eros, if you will, went off to Europe and Julie looked for another specialist.

When she shared her story with her gynecologist he was sympathetic, saying the original doctor did have a big reputation, but, as he put it, "There is no one best doctor. There are many in each field with deep experience, excellent clinical judgment, and strong communication skills."

Several of the gynecologist's patients had great success with another oncologist and he arranged for Julie to see him. Julie did and liked him for his honesty and patience with her many questions. He was willing to talk about the risks and uncertainties. She decided he was the best choice and when THE BEST OF THE BEST returned from Europe she called to say she was going elsewhere. He cemented his reputation by responding, "Of course. He's great. I'm great. Whatever."

As a case study in managing your own treatment choices there are several important elements on Julie's side. As an art dealer she was accustomed to making tough decisions based on the merits of the subject, not just the reputation. Her gynecologist had in effect a clinical trial with the doctor she chose, having sent several patients to him with success. Most important, she didn't blink. She didn't love the first one. She made a decision on the merits, not on her emotions.

How and why we pick a physician is getting more attention in the medical community from academic institutions and healthcare delivery systems, but the preferred method remains word of mouth. A relative, a friend, a family doctor, these personal connections remain the primary sources even with the vast universe of information now available in the digital age.

In 2008 the Kaiser Family Foundation looked into this and discovered that only 14 percent of patients seeking a physician saw and used the plethora of material measuring the effectiveness of care, physician expertise, and hospital standards. The Kaiser study concluded that patients are far more likely to be much more aggressive about information when buying consumer goods, such as flat-screen TVs, a computer, refrigerator, or automobile.

Younger healthcare consumers are beginning to change that. They don't hesitate to check online for comparative studies, with one survey showing just over half of the young questioned relied on physician referral while 80 percent of those sixty-five and older still prefer the doctor-to-doctor method. Younger patients also tend to have a higher level of understanding of the complexities of modern medicine.

Not surprisingly, in the vast new world of health insurance, the relationship of physicians to healthcare plans is important. The essential question: If it costs less, would you consider a narrower range of physician choices? A study of patients at four Minnesota clinics demonstrated that those buying their own insurance are overwhelmingly in favor of a smaller set of choices if it saves money. Workers with employer-provided plans were more concerned with the range of choices than the cost.

Money has always played a significant role in determining the quality of healthcare and the health of individuals. As Jesse Jackson once said during a hospital workers' strike in New York, "Rich got a plan for living. Poor got a plan for dying." The educated class knows the value of good health to quality of life and is willing to pay for it. The poor are more likely to trap themselves in a culture of smoking, poor nutrition, obesity, drugs, and only sporadic attention from a physician. Now the question is, Will the Affordable Care Act or the other forms of healthcare financial plans not only pay for treatment but educate and inspire the previously uninsured to become more responsible for their personal habits?

This cancer ordeal has reminded me again of the mental and physical dividends of good health. Every morning I awake longing for the days not so long ago when I would jump on my bike and go for a fast ride or jump in a cold mountain river for a bracing swim, walk rather than ride thirty blocks to the office. These were all habits I developed before I began making the big salaries.

Now living with the daily reality of bone pain, fatigue, the easy onset of bronchial conditions to go with the war in my veins between the powerful drugs and the villain blood cells, I have to resist self-pity and also resist the temptation of going up and down the street, shouting at construction workers to stop smoking.

I am tempted to tell them about my dad, Red, a hard-hat-wearing, lunch-bucket-carrying construction foreman who started smoking at age ten and didn't stop until he was in his fifties. He died of a heart attack at age sixty-nine.

As I was beginning my Velcade regimen, trying to adjust to a longer recovery period I walked along a Sloan corridor in the bone-marrow section and saw coming toward me a gurney occupied by a frail, gray figure, bald and hooked up to a tangle of tubes, wires, and drip bags.

We were closing fast and I wanted to say something cheerful, but as we passed I realized I couldn't tell whether the shrunken figure was a man or a woman. I tried to make eye contact but he or she was staring blankly at the passing wall, and then was gone.

I am seldom at a loss for words, but no comments in passing would be worthy.

Cancer is such a vicious disease that it can rob us of even small moments of humanity. Whatever self-pity was within me drained away. I swallowed hard, teared up, and leaned against the wall for a moment as I made my way to the Velcade start, grateful that my prognosis seemed to be better than my ghostly corridor companion's.

These cancer-patient-to-cancer-patient encounters are not unusual. A contemporary, Bill Theodore, was in treatment for lung cancer, getting his chemo through a port in his chest that allowed him to wander the hospital corridors, pushing his IV stand along. He paused to peer into a room where a much younger patient was working at a computer. The young man was gaunt, pale as an albino, and hairless. Bill heard his inner voice say, "Bill, at least you've had a life."

With the addition of Velcade to my drug diet I was scheduled to get four subcutaneous injections, one a week for a month along with my twice-a-day Revlimid dosage. It is the pharmaceutical equivalent of chemotherapy carpet bombing. Here, we hope, they are life-giving, not -taking.

The weekly Velcade injection put me back in the hands of the real worker bees of the healthcare system, the nurses. They swept into my cubicle in pairs—the Jesuit-educated daughter of a New York fireman and the young Iowan who was supporting her husband's hope of making it as a stand-up comic in New York; the expectant mother and the Long Island commuter; the willowy blonde training for the New York City Marathon.

We chatted about movies, kids, and nurse's training while they moved swiftly through the steps.

"Name and birthdate?"

"Tom Brokaw, two six four oh."

One nurse would read the code off the prescription while the other checked the match on an electronic monitor.

"Where this time, Mr. Brokaw? Abdomen?"

Yes, that seems to be working. Earlier in the day I would silently offer the veins on my left forearm for the blood extraction and testing that would determine if the Velcade could go forward.

Following kyphoplasty I felt the need for a more vigorous rehabilitation regimen, so I transferred to the Hospital for Special Surgery Sports Rehabilitation and Performance Center, internationally known for its work with world-class athletes and wannabes like me.

Polly de Mille and Rob DiGiacomo soon had me walking in a pool against an activated current, balancing on an electronic plate to determine my equilibrium, standing on a single leg to strengthen balance and muscle mass. They sent me home with instructions on how to advance my fitness on yoga mats and balance boards. I welcomed their systematic, sports-oriented approach and soon began to feel there was a chance of returning to old form.

Gratefully, Velcade seemed to work quickly. Back pain was reduced dramatically, no side effects appeared after two doses, and Meredith and I were able to join friends on Virgin Gorda, in the sunny Caribbean.

No one deserved that more than Meredith, who loves the sunshine of tropical climes. While she swam daily in the surf I waded in the pool, frustrated that my kyphoplasty prohibited one of my favorite activities, saltwater swimming. All the specialists agreed the healing had to advance before I could expose the spine to the twists required for effective stroking.

It was our first real escape from New York since September, and with an eclectic collection of companions, from rear admirals and Navy SEALs to liberal columnists and London editors, we dished and laughed and drank and ate.

Until the third day, when my office emailed that TVNewser, one of the digital sites dedicated to the serious and frivolous developments in broadcast journalism, was inquiring: "We hear Tom Brokaw has multiple myeloma and we'd like a reaction."

I had a standby response, which I swiftly transmitted to my bosses, saving a personal coda for the end. It was time. I was tired of the deception game and if it had to get out, better on my terms.

My two immediate bosses, Pat Fili-Krushel and Deborah Turness, released a statement confirming that late last summer I had been diagnosed with multiple myeloma during an examination at the Mayo Clinic.

They were generous in their description of my role at NBC News, pointing out that I had been working on a variety of NBC News projects, including the JFK documentary, making appearances on *Today*, *NBC Nightly News*, *Meet the Press*, and MSNBC as well as contributing reports to the NBC Sports coverage of the Sochi Olympics.

For my part, I said, "With the exceptional support of my family, medical team and friends, I am very optimistic about the future and look forward to continuing my life, my work and adventures still to come," adding, "I remain the luckiest guy I know," concluding with a hope that everyone would understand that I wished to keep this a private matter.

The announcement went viral, another manifestation of the desperate need of blogs and websites for material, any kind of material, especially material with a well-known name as a headline. Almost all, so far as I could tell, played it straight.

One of my home-state newspapers printed the news in "going to war"–size fonts.

Brian Williams, who had known of my condition for a while, delivered the news on his nightly broadcast from Sochi during the Winter Olympics, signaling my optimistic outlook with, "In an email tonight Tom mentioned at least the possibility of joining the Springsteen tour in Australia just to give Bruce a bump of some added publicity."

It was our small joke. I'm a fan and Brian is a close friend of The Boss.

Even with the residue of an anchorman's ego, I was unprepared for the flood tide of emails, phone calls, printed notes, and third-party good wishes and "thinking of you."

Cousins from the North Dakota branch of the Brokaws volunteered as bone marrow donors, a very difficult procedure, thankfully not required in my case. The offer alone was a welcome tonic. Friends from grade and high school checked in, some of whom I had not been in touch with for sixty years. Others dealing with MM volunteered their doctors and drug regimens.

President Obama and President Bush 41 sent notes. So did Nancy Reagan. President Clinton called, urging me to be in touch with a doctor-entrepreneurial friend who is doing breakthrough work on the genome project. Cardinal Dolan of the New York diocese wrote a warm, personal letter, saying he would remember me in his prayers. I wrote back that to be in his prayers and those of Sister Lucille Socciarelli, whom I had inherited happily from Tim Russert, would put me on a fast track.

I had a heartfelt email from Charles Barkley, the former NBA star and now basketball commentator, from his studio covering the college basketball playoffs.

We first met at a Super Bowl many years ago and he always calls me "Mr. B" and asks about children who were with me at the time.

One of the many privileges of being a national journalist for a half century is the opportunity to roam across so many parts of the American political, cultural, geographic, and socioeconomic landscape. Along the way I seemed to have made some friends, and it was emotionally gratifying to know they still feel connected to me or the work I've done. It was also reassuring to see that the ideological divides in the country can disappear under the right circumstances. In my reporting and commentary I draw fire from both ends. Yet over the years I've developed cordial professional relationships with prominent Tea Party commentators, Fox News luminaries, and outspoken pundits on the left with whom I've had disagreements. Sympathetic and welcome notes came from that wide spectrum.

One exchange that will linger: I had gone on Jon Stewart's show to promote the JFK documentary without telling Jon I was on chemo, fighting cancer. When the news came out he emailed me, "You are one tough son of a bitch."

I replied, "Jon, I didn't tell you because I didn't want to trouble you with my condition."

He wrote right back: "You can't be Jewish. I would trouble you if I had gas!"

I think that one goes in the file with the Obama, Bush, and Nancy Reagan notes.

I cherish a letter from a favorite colleague, the indestructible Sam Donaldson of ABC News. He's a cancer survivor—melanoma—and he welcomed me to the club. He recalled working with his ABC colleague Judd Rose on a cancer documentary and the question got around to "Why me?" Both were at the peak of their glamorous profession, popular and famous, highly paid, veterans of war and Washington scandal reporting. How dare cancer intervene?

An enduring story about Sam is that during a long, grueling presidential trip overseas the rest of the White House press corps was collapsed in a hotel lobby at 1:00 A.M. when Sam came charging through, throwing off commentary and needling the exhausted before retreating to his room to prepare for the day shift.

Someone asked, "What would Sam have done if they hadn't invented television?" Marty Schram of *Newsday* yawned and answered, "He would have gone door-to-door."

When familiar broadcasters write you can still hear their voice, and in his letter to me Sam's commanding style came through as he reflected on what good fortune we've both had doing what we love, and how his cancer diagnosis caused him to reflect on what he had come to take for granted.

Sam and Judd were moving from their fifties into a sixth decade. Judd settled the discussion by giving what for Sam was the only possible answer: "Why not me?"

Sam shared the story of another Washington correspondent, same age, who appeared to have terminal cancer until he went to the well-regarded Moffitt Cancer
Center in Tampa, Florida. Moffitt found a match for a
bone marrow transplant and the veteran correspondent
has gone from counting the days to enjoying a new life.
As Sam observed, there are other applications for "Why
not me?," including the bold treatment that works.

Moffitt's reputation in the world of cancer treatment
is excellent and there was a time not so long ago when
we would have known about that through physician referral or a friend's experience. Now Moffitt has a new
outlet: It is boldly advertised on the space behind the
batter's box at the televised major league games of the
Tampa Bay Rays.

Sam's letter was generous in other ways, a reminder
to me that now is the time, cancer or no cancer, to
tighten the bonds with those I care for and drift away
from those on the margins. Love as an expression of
genuine sentiment can be easily cheapened—Love ya,
babe!—but not if both parties cherish the relationship.
In notes to certain friends, male and female, I wanted
them to know that the signoff "Love" was not just a way
to end the message.

There were other reminders that my life on the merry-
go-round was slowing.

In the fall of 2013 I heard that my old colleague Garrick Utley was having serious health problems. I emailed him and didn't hear back for two weeks. Then, the jarring response. He had been homebound for two years with acute prostate cancer, drained of energy and, reading between the lines, hope. He said his wife, Gertje, a brilliant art historian, was keeping him alive. One more strong woman dedicating her life to the man she loved at a time when he needed it most.

Garrick and I were friendly generational rivals within NBC News. He broke through first, becoming Saigon bureau chief during the dominant days of *The Huntley-Brinkley Report* while I was making my way up the ladder in the California bureau. He was born to the role of journalist of the old school. His parents were both prominent Chicago journalists and active in the arts and civic affairs. Garrick studied in Europe after graduation from Carleton College and with a linguist's ear became fluent in French, German, and Russian. He developed a lifelong love of opera.

I admired his commitment to and ease in the international arena and he was among the first to congratulate me for writing *The Greatest Generation,* an extension, he said, of my feel for Main Street America. We moved in different circles socially but stayed intermittently connected until the last years of his life.

He died at age seventy-four in February 2014. When I received the call late one evening at a Mayo Clinic board meeting in Phoenix, it was not a surprise and yet I was emotionally shaken. He was one more reminder of the mortality zone I now occupy. We shared so much hope and adventure as young men and now this.

Relying on memory, I dictated an obit to the *Today* show, thinking as I would not have just a year ago, "Same age, shared experiences, good lives and then, and then . . ."

We both flourished in different spheres, coming from what I always assumed were distinctly different backgrounds. That is, until I took my mother back to her South Dakota homestead twenty years ago and visited the Conley family plot in a small cemetery along the Milwaukee Road railroad tracks that brought so many early settlers onto the prairie.

The markers with the Conley name were side by side with others bearing the name Garrick. I remarked on the coincidence to Mother and she said, "Oh, didn't I tell you? They were Garrick Utley's grandparents."

When I shared this with Garrick he was as surprised as I had been, explaining that his mother left South Dakota in the twenties to attend Stanford and then moved into the intellectual circles of Chicago.

It is an American story of westward migration and

upward mobility, from the grassland to the great events of the latter half of the twentieth century for two young men with common roots, distinctive and different upbringings, journalistic passions, and the good fortune to be in the right place at the right time.

At his memorial service I shared my first memory of him as a rising NBC News correspondent. We were told he spoke three languages and loved opera. I was unsettled by that news because I was still trying to master English and my music tastes ran more to Fats Domino, Chet Baker, and the Mamas and the Papas.

I then recalled a magical night in 1968. Meredith was with me as I was returning from a reporting trip to Europe. We stopped in Paris and Garrick invited us to dinner at a small, quintessential Parisian café on the Île de la Cité in the middle of the Seine. It was just before Christmas and when we finished the meal we emerged to a soft snowfall that might have been lifted off a canvas by Monet. Notre Dame, bathed in muted light, was at our back as we three, all of twenty-eight years old, walked back to the George V Hotel for a nightcap.

I've been to Paris many times since, often for grand occasions, but no evening will ever measure up to that one. Our ancestors buried side by side on the South Dakota prairie could not have imagined the possibilities for their grandchildren.

That shared life span made Garrick's death more emotionally difficult than I would have imagined before my own first flashing light, that computer-screen readout in a small Mayo Clinic physician's office warning of mortality.

We had the glory years and then were ambushed by the cancer years.

By the third week of February I was feeling much better, perhaps a result of the addition of the Velcade. My back pain diminished considerably, still there but more a tweak than a spasm. I was eager to get the results of a twin regimen of Velcade and the original drug, Revlimid. In one month I'd had spinal compression fractures cemented by kyphoplasty, added another high-powered chemotherapy drug, and doubled my testosterone supplement. Something should work.

First, however, Meredith had to get through her own ordeal.

Never a complainer, she had been anxious about pain in her left shoulder. An MRI revealed a substantial bone spur, and there would be no relief without surgery. After an hour in the OR, her surgeon described the spur as "epic," saying he couldn't believe she had not been complaining more. Guess he doesn't see many cowgirl-tough patients on the Upper East Side of Manhattan.

Shoulder injuries and repairs are notoriously aggravating, making it difficult to sleep, or to get through a day. The patient is almost permanently hooked up to an icing machine for the first week.

In typical stoic fashion Meredith soldiered on with some help from me and our longtime home manager, the estimable Goldine Nicholas. We attached Meredith to the icing machine and helped arrange the sleeping conditions, stood back, and waited for the complaints related to what every shoulder injury veteran says is deep pain.

Not a whimper, except when I accidently bumped her wounds while changing a dressing. She quietly threatened to have me replaced.

That would not do. I needed the job mostly because I needed to be with her, always, in whatever condition.

I began telling callers we were running a MASH unit without the benefit of Alan Alda's sardonic wit.

There were some advantages. Confined to quarters, planning the evening meal became a more elaborate process. Deciding what to watch—*House of Cards* on Netflix or a DVD of *12 Years a Slave* as a warmup for the Oscars telecast.

Spending more time in front of the television set gave me new insights into mass marketing. First, no one in any commercial seems to be unhappy or angry, whatever the circumstances. A neighbor trimming a tree drops a huge limb onto your car parked in your driveway, totally wrecking it. In real life the car owner would go ballistic, reaching for a baseball bat to give chase to the chainsaw misfit, screaming obscenities. Or he'd show up with a platoon of lawyers prepared to sue the neighbor for everything he has.

But in TV Commercial–land, the aggrieved party is next seen with a friendly insurance agent, smiling happily about what he is sure will be a swift and appropriate settlement.

Right.

If obesity is a national epidemic, has anyone calculated the number of calories represented in a day of fastfood commercials? It is one gut bomb after another, dripping with layers of bacon, cheese, ground beef, fried jalapeño peppers, cheerily consumed by slim models who treat these caloric megatons as if they were an aphrodisiac.

I am not a food scold. I believe in individual choice, not mandated restrictions, but if the liquor and beer companies are expected to remind consumers about responsible drinking, if advertisements for over-thecounter or prescription drugs are required to list all the possible side effects, why not expect fast-food companies to list the calories in the sandwiches they advertise as if they are the elixir of life?

As for me, slowly, my appetite began to return, but I am determined to keep the extra weight off even though the new wardrobe and alterations are not incidental expenses. I try for a hearty oatmeal breakfast and a cocktail of lemonade, orange juice, and cranberry juice to attack the drug-induced dehydration. I can handle a partial cocktail or most of a glass of red wine but no more than that.

Day after day, friends are saying, "How you doing? By the way, you look GREAT!"

Huh? I look better *with* cancer than I did without?

When the news of my condition was broadcast it earned me a new wave of friends and strangers alike who offered physician references and family histories of MM. Once they hear the makeup of my new team their own doctors generally say, "He's got the right doctors doing the right thing."

The personal case histories were the most encouraging. A prominent Los Angeles public relations executive has been living with MM for fourteen years, rides horses, and has an altogether active life on drug maintenance. An Arizona man survived MM and with his wife set up a foundation and website for other families bewildered by the diagnosis.

I learned, for the first time, that Frank McGee, host

of the *Today* show from 1971 to 1974, suffered from MM and kept it from everyone despite his ever more gaunt appearance. When he died after putting in another full week on the air his producers and friends were stunned.

Sam Walton, founder of Walmart, was another MM casualty, which led many to believe that he had established the high-profile multiple myeloma treatment center in Little Rock, Arkansas. This is a full-immersion process in which MM is the singular target under the commanding title of Myeloma Institute for Research and Therapy. There is a Walton auditorium on the institute's University of Arkansas medical school campus, but the institute itself was founded by Bart Barlogie, a renowned MM specialist from the MD Anderson Cancer Center in Houston.

The institute has an impressive record, running well ahead of the national average for survival for those who are dealing with MM. One number is especially notable. The institute has followed 1,070 patients for more than ten years, and 783 have never had a relapse of the disease.

Sam Walton was treated by Dr. Barlogie at MD Anderson before the Little Rock institute was founded, but the connection ended there. Walton, who'd had an earlier struggle with leukemia, didn't survive his encounter with multiple myeloma, dying in April 1992, a time when life expectancy for a man his age with this cancer was short.

I was unaware of all of this when I was diagnosed. I took comfort in the repeated reassurances of specialists that great progress in treating MM with a new class of drugs, your own body's reengineered immunology system, was rapidly improving chances of a longer survival than the published five to ten years.

As I began to respond to treatment the favored and welcome line was, "You're gonna die but from something else."

Spring

By early April I was feeling stronger than at any time since the diagnosis. Ron Olson, my fellow Mayo board member and the first to know, called on a Saturday evening to get a report and I said, "Best I've felt in a long while."

Sunday morning I awoke feeling "fluie," an expression favored by Meredith's doctor father at the onset of flu. By that evening it went from onset to full-blown. I was miserable with congestion, aches in other muscles, swallowing difficulties.

With germ-fighting blood cells on the other team a flu infection can quickly go terminal. So for only the second time in my life I was quickly rolling down a Sloan corridor in a wheelchair, headed for treatment against this potentially perilous condition.

Once again at the check-in: "Tom Brokaw, two six four oh."

The Sloan urgent care physician in charge asked on entry if I'd had a flu shot. Of course, just last September. "So did I," she explained, "but I'm just back after eight days out with this strain. I think our flu shots were for last year's flu."

There it is again, the body's constant adaptation to help or hurt us, the vast, intricate systems reacting to whatever enters their spheres of influence.

Scientists in the lab and physicians in their practices are learning more every day about the connectivity of this universe of parts and fluids and still they have untold miles to go, stopping and starting for clinical trials, new imaging devices and investigations into the sources of new, dangerous conditions that pop up every day.

My spacious room quickly became a ward of its own.

Saline solution drips, antibiotics every six hours, teams of internal medicine specialists and their residents, pulmonologists with breathing aids, nurses, and Jennifer, who flew in from Nashville, where she had been for a friend's fiftieth birthday.

Two nights, three days of intense, round-the-clock care and I was able to return home with the cautionary warning that I seemed to be susceptible to bronchial episodes and it would require close monitoring.

As every hospital visit seemed to, this one turned up another memorable immigrant story. One of the young pulmonologists had an engaging personality so I probed some. He was Chinese.

Medical school? I asked.

He chuckled, "Beijing but also Taipei; I'm Taiwanese but I was educated in Belize."

What?

He explained that when he was ten his father, the proprietor of a modest Taiwanese restaurant, saw a video promising to teach Chinese kids English in Belize in six months. So the dad sent my new friend to Belize at age ten with his slightly older brother and there they stayed for eight years, learning English and a good deal more.

They returned home on long, circuitous flights for summers and then went back to Belize. Steven Hsu said his parents were what the Chinese call "tiger parents," very demanding, and he adored them for making him what he is today. When the family restaurant had some economic difficulties he and his wife, a bank analyst, bought his parents a bed and breakfast in Belize.

I think I'll visit them on my next fishing trip to that tiny English-speaking enclave.

I was dismissed and sent home with medications and breathing aids to temper the bronchial conditions. My bathroom was beginning to resemble a pharmaceutical discount store.

.   .   .

When spring arrived I remembered that initial autumn visit to Sloan and the physician who assured me that by spring I would be up and running around. I don't feel like running around. I'd settle for just one day of feeling great.

The warmer weather and longer sunny days were welcome but they also tried my patience. Walking our dog, Red, in Central Park, I was moving slowly, looking, I'm sure, like an old man out for a stroll before a 5:30 supper at a local diner and an early bedtime. A handsome, athletic couple, probably in their early forties, bounded into the park off Fifth Avenue and began loosening up for a jog.

Fleetingly, I was tempted to say, "Hey, that was me once, I didn't always look like this."

Instead I simply continued on my route, trying to put a little more bounce in my shuffle in case they were watching.

Sunday mornings north of Manhattan, in bucolic Westchester County, were especially difficult. Meredith would drive to a Starbucks and get the Sunday papers while I sat in the passenger side, staring out at the string of bicyclists pedaling furiously along the tree-lined streets, past the stately homes with the manicured flower beds now in bloom, and around the reservoirs. That was me a year ago and I so took it for granted that I am now self-critical for not fully appreciating the privilege.

.   .   .

The chemo carpet bombing continued and I was fortunate not to have an adverse reaction.

The morning President Obama dedicated the evocative National September 11 Memorial Museum in lower Manhattan I was asked to join Matt Lauer and Savannah Guthrie for a special *Today* interruption to cover the event.

"Tom Brokaw, two six four oh."

I agreed without telling them I would arrange my drug treatment at an earlier time so I could meet their schedule.

Matt and I had been side by side for the first hours of the 9/11 attacks so it was in a way a continuum and it seemed to go well, as we described the contemporary scene and recalled that dreadful morning, especially the collapse of the towers.

When I am asked about the most challenging stories of my career the attacks of 9/11 are at the top of the breaking news category. The collapse of the Soviet Union and the redefinition of Communist China will be more historically important and transformative.

On that September morning in 2001 I had just finished an exhausting yoga session, my first, when the phone rang. Small plane. World Trade Center. Better come in.

Leaving our apartment I heard the sirens of trucks from our neighborhood firehouse as a caravan of big red outfits headed crosstown to the West Side Highway for the escorted trip to the World Trade Center.

For most of Manhattan, it was otherwise a clear, beautiful morning, election day for a mayoral primary. Running for a cab, I asked a neighbor if he had heard the news. Confused, he said, "The election is not over already, is it?"

Within minutes that confused innocence gave way to a horrific reality. In the cab I heard a well-known radio news reporter describe the second plane flying low over Washington Square Park and into tower number one.

What the hell is going on?

I awoke Meredith in Montana, told her to turn on the television, and said, "I don't know when we'll be able to talk again."

Matt Lauer and Katie Couric were on duty on the *Today* show set as I slid in beside them, beginning the single most challenging day of my career. This was a monumental event for which we had no warning: men flying hijacked civilian airliners into towering symbols of American wealth and enterprise, television screens filling with eerie images of smoky plumes enveloping the upper floors of the towers, the knowledge that fifty thousand people were at work in those offices when the attack came.

Scattered reports from little-known Middle Eastern organizations claiming credit began to trickle in. Our

Washington bureau chief, Tim Russert, was working the phones hard, trying to determine how many other airliners might have been hijacked, when we were interrupted by Jim Miklaszewski, NBC's Pentagon correspondent. He reported a loud boom and a shudder through the building from the west side of the Pentagon. The headquarters of America's military might had been attacked by another hijacked airliner, American Airlines Flight 77.

Meanwhile, we kept the cameras fixed on the twin towers, the monolithic steel and glass structures reaching 110 stories into the sky from the foot of Wall Street, plumes of smoke and fire billowing out from their high floors. The images were captured on a long-range lens so it was a silent, almost serene scene, utterly misrepresentative of the chaos at ground zero and in the buildings.

How many got safely out?

And how many were forced to jump to escape the fires? Those images began to fleetingly appear—a couple holding hands as they plummeted, a woman fluttering her arms. I am incapable, even now, all these years later, of finding words that do justice to my emotions.

Almost instantly there was an agreement to not televise these desperate scenes.

As the fires continued I said aloud, "There is so much structural damage these towers will have to be brought down," and instantly regretted my comment. What did I know? Maybe they could survive.

Moments later tower two began its sickening collapse, slow at first and then a rush to a monumental storm of debris and death. We had no idea how many still were trapped inside.

In all the years I've been anchoring live events—the start of wars, election nights, inaugurations, natural disasters, space shots and space disasters—there had never been anything like this. A deliberate suicidal attack on two of the tallest office buildings in the world, bringing them down with an unknown number of deaths.

After the second tower collapsed, a slow-motion death spiral, I felt compelled to say on the air, "This will change us in ways we cannot yet anticipate."

And then, looking steadily into the camera, I declared, "We're at war."

Thirteen years later we're in our third war as a result of rage in the name of Islam, still trying to find a military and political strategy for defeating an uncommon enemy, fueled by a maniacal devotion to destroy Western culture in the name of preserving and expanding a deeply radical view of Islam.

It is a war of great complexity, including Muslim against Muslim, in which the enemy is highly mobile in a forbidding landscape, financed by private, shadowy wealth from within our allies, including Saudi Arabia and Qatar.

How it ends is unclear. There will be no surrender ceremonies on a U.S. battleship, no new Islamic state constrained by its neighbors and monitored by Western military forces.

How do you conquer the fanatic who answers only to his own distortion of a great and ancient faith?

On all my trips to the region I invariably encounter these kinds of exchanges, in a souk, a coffeehouse, on a street corner. A young Iraqi male will approach and ask, "Are you an American?" Yes. The response? "I love America, but if you harm one hair on my sister's head I will join jihad against you!" It may be a Shia opposed to Sunni rule, but America's actions can bind them in common cause.

If only the cancer of Islamic fratricide were subject to the drugs that were my allies in fighting multiple myeloma.

My personal well-being depends on the genius of pharmacologists and other laboratory technicians to develop test-tube weapons for the war raging in my body between cancerous and healthy blood cells. While they are working long hours into the night to advance the quality of human life, Islamic despots pillage, rape, and behead their way across Muhammad's land in a frenzy of violence right out of the Middle Ages.

·   ·   ·

When the 2014 special report ended thirteen years after the initial attacks I said to Matt, "Well, it's been a full morning. Ninety minutes ago I was getting pumped through with chemo drugs and from there to this." He was briefly wide-eyed and then typically solicitous, saying when this is all over we'll get in some golf.

Because of the spinal issues golf is off the schedule for now, and maybe for a long time.

Before the diagnosis my back pain became so severe during an annual outing with then New York City mayor Mike Bloomberg I had to be driven off the course.

We're a couple of duffers constantly trying to get better and we have an annual match for a quarter a hole (Bloomberg claims that's how he became a billionaire). At the time I had to leave the course Mike was up two holes. So now I say, "Rather than lose to the mayor, I developed cancer."

In the spring of 2014 I was sitting at my desk when an email arrived from Jennifer. Brother Bill was failing fast. He could no longer swallow. He developed apnea, a stoppage of breathing, requiring twenty-four-hour monitoring, and he seemed to have just given up, spending most of his time in bed. Jennifer guessed he had a week at best.

She told the hospice nurse, "No heroic measures; his body is signaling his time is up."

I burst into tears, unexpectedly, because although I knew the moment was coming he'd been my brother for seventy-one years.

Everything that seemed to go right in my life went the other way for Bill and I've always had an emotional hangover as a result. Unfairly, how many times did he have a teacher say, "Tom was one of my best," or, later, "Tom Brokaw's brother? What's that like?"

Now we were both sick but I am going to get better and he isn't.

Through my tears I spotted a crib we had erected in our New York apartment for a visit from Archer, Sarah's son. Before his steep decline, Uncle Bill had never failed to smile when recalling Sarah's visit with Archer.

These are the cycles of life. We lose a member of a family and another comes along to renew the continuity, a chain of death and birth that has been under way since the arrival of upright man.

Staring at the crib, remembering Archer's peaceful nap a short while ago, gave me solace, as I hoped it would Bill in some metaphysical way. It reminded me of what Sarah had said earlier, when I was lamenting what an ugly year it had been for the Brokaws.

"Dad!" she said. "Don't forget, we had Archer. He made it a GREAT year."

She was right, of course. This precious addition is a tribute to the ever-evolving place and rewards of family.

Bill died a few days later, in the company of Denver friends and his hospice nurse. There were flashes of the old Bill right to the end. He was sleeping most of the time and when he awoke one morning in his final week his nurse said, "You looked happy. Were you dreaming?"

"Yes," he replied.

"Dreaming of what?" she asked.

"Women," he said with a small smile.

We knew he was ready to let go when he told Jennifer he wanted to see Red, which was the name of our Labrador, named after my father.

Jennifer, thinking he meant the dog, said, "But, Bill, he's in Montana."

"No," he protested. "Red, my dad."

"He's in heaven," Jennifer said. "You want to go there?"

"Yeah," he replied.

His death was sad but a relief and, in its own way, welcome for all. He was free of this dreadful disease and the family members were free of nagging questions. "Am I doing enough?"

Jennifer need not have asked the question. Her tough love as the daughter he never had was a model. In the midst of all this she wrote an essay for *Time* magazine in which she argued that the women's movement needs to address the disproportionate place of women as caregivers in our aging society, too often at the expense of their careers and personal health.

Alzheimer's is a disease profoundly personal in its arc from normal to mental, physical, and psychological dysfunctional behavior. It is the immediate family that knows best the depth of destruction and pays the price emotionally.

While researchers race to find a cure and entrepreneurs finance the construction of more assisted living facilities, middle-aged children should be expected to look at their aging parents and wonder: "Are we next? If we are, how do we pay for it, handle it emotionally, and what will it do to the quality of our own lives?"

Bill's passing and my cancer were another intersection in our lives in which it worked out better for me. As we prepared to lose him I had an appointment to assess the results of the more aggressive treatment. It was the most important evaluation since the diagnosis and I was low-grade anxious. I like to have an idea of the outcome, whatever the experience. Besides, I was increasingly aware of the good days I was giving up. At my age they're not easily recaptured.

"Tom Brokaw, two six four oh."

Meredith and I arrived early at Dr. Landau's examination room, riffling through the email and personal projects on our iPads. Heather walked in with her typically pleasant but low-key greeting, leaned up against the examination table, and said, "Well, it's good news. The tumor in the soft tissue around the pelvis has disappeared." (Did I know there had been a tumor in the soft tissue? I was so concentrated on blood and bones, I don't think so.) Going on, she read from her notes, "The bones are healing and getting stronger. The blood count has improved significantly. It is very close to where we want it."

Silently, I thought, Yes! Maybe there is an endgame to all of this after all.

The chemotherapy would continue through the summer and she wanted to add gamma globulin therapy as a defense against those recurring bronchial conditions.

By fall, she said, there was a good chance I could move to a drug maintenance program, which is what gives MM patients most of their life back.

Thank you, Revlimid, Velcade, and dexamethasone, my old friends, I look forward to seeing you again.

Dr. Anderson at Dana-Farber and Dr. Gertz at Mayo were equally pleased. Whatever differences they had in treatment, the results were impressive. At breakfast with Dr. Gertz he used the encomium "spectacular" as he left the table.

After sharing the good news with family and friends I

typically overreached with spring and summer plans. The new U.S. ambassador to Italy, John Phillips, and his wife, former CBS correspondent Linda Douglass, invited me the first weekend in June to discuss the Italian campaign during World War II and the fall of Rome, which came one day before D-Day in Normandy and thus was largely lost to history.

Why not? Bronchitis again, that's why not. It would not clear in time for Rome and there was some question whether I could get to Normandy for the seventieth anniversary of D-Day. NBC News had made extensive plans.

After a militarylike assault on the bronchitis I was cleared for the flight to England. Meredith and I joined a fund-raising cruise organized by the National World War II Museum in New Orleans, the impressive and still-expanding tribute to that seminal event in American life.

When the late historian Stephen Ambrose first envisioned and then began construction on the museum, it was to commemorate D-Day and the landing craft that had made the invasion possible. They were Higgins boats, designed and built by Andrew Higgins in New Orleans.

Steven Spielberg and Tom Hanks of *Saving Private Ryan* and I helped launch the museum with donations and personal appearances. We continued after Ambrose's death when his fellow historian Gordon H. "Nick" Mueller took over and agreed to expand the mission to a museum of the whole war, not just the invasion. It has become a national treasure, with several wings containing tanks, fighter planes, bombers, virtual reality submarine missions, oral histories, and an IMAX film produced by Hanks that leaves viewers breathless.

For the cruise Mueller booked several prominent World War II historians, including Rick Atkinson, who lectured nightly and provided commentary during tours of the key D-Day sites. As the amateur in the class I concentrated on the personal stories of ordinary men without whom the invasion would have failed.

I reminded the guests that the invasion had succeeded not just because of the brave infantrymen who waded ashore, and the paratroopers who jumped behind enemy lines, but also because of the medics who were constantly exposed to enemy fire as they desperately tried to save the lives of gravely wounded soldiers crying out for help or, as everyone there that day remembers, crying out for their mothers. And then there were the graves registration teams that came ashore to collect dog tags from the mortally wounded so they could be identified. The young men wrestling trucks and half-tracks onto the beach to keep the supply lines open.

I told them about Frank DeVita, with whom I had spent the day on Omaha Beach with thirty members of his family. Frank had dropped out of high school to enlist in the Coast Guard when war broke out, and on June 6, 1944, he was an eighteen-year-old gunner's mate on the USS *Samuel Chase*. He was ordered to leave his gun position and man the forward ramp on a landing craft headed onto Omaha under heavy enemy fire.

Seventy years later Frank remembered:

When we got near the beach one particular machine gun took a liking to us and was hitting my boat, [making a sound] like a typewriter.

The Germans had the high ground and were shooting down at us. It was like hitting fish in a barrel.

My job was to drop the ramp and I knew in my head—even though I was a young kid—when I drop the ramp, instead of the bullets hitting the ramp they would come into the boat. So the coxswain says, "Drop the ramp," and I made believe I didn't hear him.

So he said it a second time and again I made believe I didn't hear him. Third time he says, "Goddammit, DeVita, drop the effing ramp."

So we had thirty men on the boat. Three men

made it to the beach. They were all wounded and some of them were dead.

DeVita can still hear their cries. "You know, there's a fallacy, people think that when a man is dying. . . . They don't ask for God. The last word that they say before they die is 'Mama, mama.'"

As Frank and I stood on Omaha seventy years later he was surrounded by his family, his wife, children, and grandchildren. As he remembered that day and the life he was able to have, denied to those who fell when the ramp went down, we both choked up and he said, "These kids were eighteen, nineteen years old. They're never gonna see their sons play Little League baseball. They're never gonna walk their daughter down the aisle. And they're never gonna hold their grandchild in their arms."

After an emotional farewell to the DeVita family I made my way awkwardly across the sands of Omaha Beach and around the pools of rainwater, still favoring my painful back and weakened legs but thinking, "This will end. We've got cancer on the run. I get to hold my grandchildren."

By the end of that week, I had spent time with a member of the 82nd Airborne who jumped into Normandy, a pilot who flew paratroopers across the channel, and a Rhode Island veteran on his first trip back after a horrendous landing seventy years earlier. He was a member of a navy explosive assault team and the first off their rubber raft as it hit the beach. A moment later the raft took a direct hit and all his teammates were killed. He was left to wonder, as so many D-Day survivors do, "Why was I spared?"

Deborah Turness suggested I find the words and images to sum up the week. This is what I wrote and Brian Williams and the NBC *Nightly News* team broadcast:

(sound of muted taps in the background)
(scenes of headstones—individual and row upon row)

"This is why we're here," I said softly. "Here above the beaches of Normandy,"

(sound of surf)

"just beyond the water"

(incoming surf)

"that brought liberty—at a great sacrifice."

(faces of D-Day vets)

"For those who survived that day and so many others this is a journey of honor and remembrance.
"To honor their fallen friends and remember, seventy years later."

(ceremony)

"But it is not just the veterans who honor the sacrifices here."

(Obama and company)

"A new generation of leaders takes up the call."

OBAMA: We tell the story for the old soldiers who pull themselves a little straighter today to salute brothers who never made it home. We tell the story for the daughter who clutches a faded photo of her father, forever young. . . .

Gentlemen, I want each of you to know that your legacy is in good hands.

"And the President reminded us that their legacy goes beyond the fighting to the costly time to their young lives."

OBAMA: They left home barely more than boys and returned home heroes. But to their great credit, that is not how this generation carried itself. After the war some put away their medals, were quiet about their service, moved on.

(Brokaw voice-over)

"But before they could go home there was Normandy.
"There had never been anything like it before and there would never be again.

"Now in their late eighties and nineties, so many of these veterans will not be around for the seventy-fifth anniversary."

(*vet in wheelchair*)

"Their lives are coming to a close."

(*bring in taps*)

"But their legacy can never be dimmed."

That essay—words, images, and sounds—was the opening of NBC *Nightly News with Brian Williams* that night and it was for me a distillation of all my experiences on these sacred sands and beachheads. Normandy is now a part of my life in a way I could never have known it would become when I first arrived more than thirty years ago.

I've heard the American presidents speak—Reagan, Clinton, Bush 43, Obama—and watched the families embrace the survivors, I've told the stories of heroism and loss, witnessed the twenty-one-gun salutes and the playing of the anthems. In the final hours of each of these anniversaries I am reminded again that these tributes, however grand, are inadequate to commemorate what happened here. As long as there is recorded history D-Day will be remembered as a monumental triumph of

freedom over oppression won by military audacity carried ashore by men and boys who died, lost their limbs,
survived, and gave us all an enduring lesson in the virtues of humble valor.

I was exhausted by the end of the week but I would
not have been anywhere else.

Summer

Returning to New York I began to plot the summer.

Could it have been just a year ago that the onset of back pain was aggravating, a nuisance I thought would quickly clear up once I got the right exercises? Once the cancer diagnosis was established, Meredith and the physicians counseled patience, saying, "Next year at this time you'll be much better."

It is now close to "next year at this time" and I am better but I am not yet sturdy enough to wade rivers running even moderately high and fast. The daily dose of high-powered drugs drains energy, and as I compensate for aches on one side of my back, new ones appear on the other. Will I have a trouble-free, back-to-normal day anytime soon, or is this the new life of a man who is old in body and spirit?

Those spirits were lifted by a unique summer reunion on a series of bluffs along the south-central South Dakota stretch of the Missouri River, home of the stately Fort Randall Dam, a massive public works project initiated immediately after World War II.

When my family arrived in the area in 1947 it was a nineteenth-century tableau of an abandoned cavalry fort, a few Yankton Sioux Indian homes along the river bottom, and a few small towns nearby to serve the farming community.

The U.S. Army Corps of Engineers were in charge of building a new town to house the thousands of workers needed to complete the ten-year project, the largest earth-rolled dam of its kind in the United States.

Within two years the corps had constructed a modern town with graceful boulevards, shopping center, state-of-the-art high school, hospital, movie theater, hotel, recreation center, and a mix of triplexes, duplexes, single-family homes, and trailer lots for more than three thousand residents who came as welders, electricians, truck drivers, operators of enormous excavation machinery, ironworkers, carpenters, engineers, and surveyors.

They were from the Midwest, the Deep South, the Southwest, and California, refugees from the Great Depression and veterans of World War II. This was their first real opportunity to make a good wage, buy a car, think about sending a son or daughter to college.

The Brokaws moved into a three-bedroom duplex with hardwood floors and an up-to-date kitchen, easily the best housing my parents had ever occupied. Dad bought his first new car and Mother got a deep freeze.

The southerners brought hush puppies and soft drawls, Okies had two names—Bobby Gene—and the midwestern crowd taught all how to hunt pheasants and fish the Missouri. It was a working-class nirvana and ten years later it was over. The dam was completed, the town folded up, and we all moved on, with lingering memories of the good times.

A few years ago some of the high school graduates who went on to become engineers, orthopedists, physicians, developers, businessmen, decided a small museum was in order to remind everyone what had gone on there.

I produced a ten-minute minidocumentary and the organizing committee did an impressive job of displaying photos, artifacts, construction plans, and local Indian lore. Five hundred people showed up, including some of my most cherished boyhood friends. One, my regular camping tent mate, still had his irreverent sense of humor, confiding he tells his Minnesota small-town friends when they ask if he knew me, "Know him? Hell, I slept with him."

The weekend was a snapshot of a time gone by, the can-do years right after the war when national pride and optimism were the twin drivers of the American Dream.

Families arrived in aged cars, some from homes with

no indoor plumbing, to find their first steady job at a good wage. They left in new vehicles, money in the bank and kids ready for college.

The reunion weekend received heavy local press coverage. My old friends, most of whom I had not seen in more than half a century, were relieved that I was on the mend. One, from a large Irish American family, was a classmate who lost his mother to cancer. I remember her ghostly appearance when I'd visit their home, which had a funereal air as she made her way slowly from room to room. It was a haunting experience and when I recalled it, Jerry paused and said, "I was just nine."

Those were the days when the word "cancer" was rarely uttered in public, as if the sound alone was some kind of a curse. Now at large benefit dinners to fund cancer research survivors are asked to stand, magazines feature the latest treatments and offer suggestions on how to cope, obituaries have adopted the phrase "courageous battle" to describe cancer victims' final days.

Before returning to Montana I made a pilgrimage to Cooperstown, New York, for a baseball fan's religious ceremony: the induction of a new class of major league legends.

It was a legendary class. Pitchers Tom Glavine and Greg Maddux of the Atlanta Braves; power hitter Frank

Thomas of the Chicago White Sox; managers Joe Torre of the Yankees, Tony La Russa of the Cardinals, and Bobby Cox of the Braves.

In an era of mega-events, Hall of Fame weekend is a restoration of a time gone by in small-town America, with sports heroes and their families thrilled to be selected, sharing bus rides and golf games, parades down Cooperstown's Main Street, and after-dinner drinks in the bars of the Otesaga Hotel, a grand old resort on Lake Otsego.

My ticket to the weekend was a foreword I wrote for the hall's seventy-fifth anniversary memorial book, a handsomely designed publication featuring photographs and baseball descriptions of every player in the shrine.

Fred Wilpon, the owner of the New York Mets, and his wife, Judith, gave me a ride to Cooperstown on their plane and made sure I was on the inside of the weekend's rituals. That included dinner with Fred's friend since their days as teenage teammates, the incomparable Sandy Koufax. Sandy was in the last year of his Hall of Fame career with the Los Angeles Dodgers when I moved to Southern California, and often when he pitched I tried to be in the press box so I could have a straight look at his overpowering fastball and breaking pitches. Not for the first time, I had a full appreciation of those who say the most difficult task in sports is hitting a ball thrown at eighty to ninety miles an hour from sixty feet away—a ball breaking down or away at the plate, and your only weapon is a thirty-six-ounce tubular piece of ash.

Now seventy-eight, Koufax remains a handsome, trim man, still carrying himself with an easy reserve in his tailored blazer and tie—always a tie throughout the weekend. We'd met a couple of times before and I was flattered he remembered me from my Los Angeles days, partly because, he said, laughing, "Your tie knot was always crooked."

Damn! He was right. In my first year on the air I tied an ugly knot, never knowing that Sandy Koufax was looking on. I corrected it later but having Koufax remember it almost fifty years later gives it a certain panache.

Having dinner with Koufax, high-fiving Johnny Bench and Reggie Jackson, both of whom I've known for a while, trading Omaha stories with Bob Gibson, laughing—again—at Tommy Lasorda stories, a morning chat with Cal Ripken on the picturesque hotel veranda, congratulating Glavine and La Russa in the hotel lobby, hanging out with Billy Crystal, a guest of Joe Torre's, catching up with Hank Aaron, with whom I did a documentary about his successful quest to break Babe Ruth's home run record—well, it was good to be excused from cancer for a while.

Reality returned Sunday afternoon during the out-door ceremonies. The afternoon began with a familiar sound carrying across the expansive grass amphitheater, as jumbo screens carried the poetic MLB Network opening for the induction. Bob Costas had suggested me as the narrator and I was happy to be somehow involved, if only as a voice.

The Wilpons secured third-row seats for the ceremony, which had all the appearance of a reunion of a college championship team until you looked more closely. There's George Brett, Mike Schmidt, Brooks Robinson, Phil Niekro, Barry Larkin, Frank Robinson, Carlton "Pudge" Fisk, Juan Marichal, Gaylord Perry, Tom Seaver, Nolan Ryan—a stage full of certified baseball immortals.

I knew it would be a long afternoon and worried about my stamina. Sitting in the sun, a fresh dose of chemo running through my system, I faded, fast. The Wilpons, alert to my discomfort and so attentive all weekend, were quick to get me to an air-conditioned holding room, where I stretched out for a restorative sleep. I awoke for the closing speeches, but after such a magical time I wanted nothing more than to return to New York and my own bed.

Damn this cancer. How dare it interfere with such a glorious time?

. . .

What was that World War I saying, "Trust the Lord and pass the ammo"?

For me, trust the doctors and the Lord and pass the Velcade, Revlimid, dexamethasone.

In August I was headed back to Rochester for a Mayo public trustees meeting, one year after my initial diagnosis at the clinic. Morie Gertz, who made the initial call, and Andrew Majka, my perceptive primary care physician who suspected myeloma, met me in front of a computer screen and started scrolling the results.

In one measurement after another my condition from a year ago showed a mark far above normal and then a steady, precipitous fall to intersect or touch the flat line of normalcy. Dr. Gertz checked them off in his usual brusque fashion: "See this? From heavy involvement a year ago a steady drop to kiss the flat line of normal."

Dr. Gertz went from "You have a malignancy" a year ago to the welcome conclusion, "The myeloma is gone."

Whew! Now what? I have learned to leaven my reactions with the realities of what may come next. In this case, it was time to begin thinking about the next step, maintenance therapy.

Doctors Landau and Anderson agreed the numbers were impressive, but they elected to finish another round of chemo to nail a protein issue. It was not yet time to get out the Gatorade bucket to soak the medical team and accept the trophy but we were getting close.

I still had much more back pain than I wanted. Nonetheless, as I told family and friends, "The light at the end of the tunnel just got much larger."

From Rochester I flew to Denver for brother Bill's memorial. We decided to have only immediate family gather in a leafy enclave alongside a remote stream northwest of Denver. Mike and I shared some reminiscences of brotherly brawling and family feuds that were more hilarious than serious and over almost before they began.

Having spent most of our childhood on the Missouri River on the Great Plains, I've always been drawn to the metaphorical qualities of rivers. Here I said, "Streams and rivers are like life—they have a source and a destination. They have stretches of calmness and turmoil. No day on the river is ever exactly the same, as it is not in life."

Then Dan Foster, a second cousin by marriage, waded into the stream and committed Bill's ashes to the current, where they left a discernible white trail before quickly dissolving.

We linked arms and our eldest granddaughter, Claire, led the small circle of family members in a soft, a cappella rendition of "Amazing Grace." For Bill's favorite cousin, Angie, it was a deeply felt moment as she closed her eyes tight and swayed to the familiar lyrics.

Amazing grace, how sweet the sound.
That saved a wretch like me.
I once was lost but now I'm found.
Was blind, but now I see.

Following the streamside service we gathered care-givers and close friends for a hearty Tex-Mex lunch in Morrison, a quaint touristy village just north of the Red Rocks outdoor concert hall.

Mike, cousin Dick, and Ben, Bill's stepson, quickly got into Bill's sneaky habit of exhibiting the middle-finger salute in almost every family photograph—a down-market version of the famed theatrical artist Al Hirschfeld working his daughter Nina's name into every sketch.

I recalled that twenty minutes before I walked down the aisle to marry Meredith with Bill and Mike as groomsmen, Mother called us all together, including Dad, and said, "It comes to an end right here, right now."

We didn't have to ask what "it" she had in mind. We followed orders.

As the luncheon proceeded, various caregivers arose to pay tribute to Bill and his curious combination of sweetness, ornery charm, and quirky sense of humor.

Pete, a gregarious bus driver for the facility, described Bill's concern for a small rabbit living in a drainpipe outside his room. He checked on him on winter mornings and made sure food was left out. Pete was aware of Bill's fondness for pets, especially a beautiful Irish setter, Tag, who was the child he never had.

So Pete excitedly described the day toward Bill's end when he brought in his Labradoodle puppy and placed the small dog on Bill's bed. As he tried to describe Bill's joy, Pete's eyes filled and he couldn't go on for some time.

Rorry, another caregiver, repeated the story about dreaming and women, laughing and crying at the typical Bill mischievous humor, surfacing as it did just a few days before he died.

These are heroic people, the staffs of assisted living facilities, dealing every day for modest wages with patients who mentally occupy a bizarre universe of failed neural synapses giving way to forgetfulness, loss of language, and incapacity for the most fundamental mental and physical tasks, including body functions.

Back in Montana, following Bill's service, I began to expand my physical fitness routines with longer walks and longer wades in the West Boulder River, which bisects our property. Wading against the current is a test even for the physically fit but I was determined to use nature's gift as a strengthening source. I used a wading staff for balance and despite the worries of my physicians I did not fall.

When not in the river, I pushed through waist-high grass with Red, my Labrador, hoping to locate coveys of Hungarian partridge or sharp-tailed grouse, keeping an eye out for rattlesnakes, pausing to watch our robust population of antelope do their ballet across the open fields.

Our property is at 5,600 feet, so the altitude combined with the difficult terrain is an aid for fitness. It is also a reminder of just how much I had "deconditioned," to use a word favored by one of my therapists. I tired after a forty-minute walk in the hills or a hundred-yard wade against the current.

Two summers ago a friend thirty years younger and I climbed a steep, rocky peak laced with deadfall—trees that had given up to snow and wind—by bushwhacking through the treacherous terrain that had no trail. It was a six-hour trek up and down but I had no residual aches and pains. Maybe I'll be ready for a similar challenge in my seventy-fifth summer. Right now I'd settle for a two-hour stretch in the river with no streamside naps.

Before I get there I have a pesky blood marker to get under control. It's called M spike, one of the distinctive signs of myeloma. It is a gathering of malignant plasma cells in the same place. It has been greatly reduced, but

Doctors Landau and Anderson want to reduce it to zero—so they've ordered at least two more cycles of chemotherapy.

Meanwhile, I'm feeling markedly better. The fact that I have cancer is no longer a twenty-four-hour presence in my consciousness. The cancer screen through which I viewed the world is now a faint presence. Friends remark on my stronger voice and physical erectness.

I began to feel well enough to reignite my travel schedule and plunge into the documentary I agreed to do on Angelina Jolie's making of *Unbroken* as a feature film. She was deeply affected, as so many of us were, by Laura Hillenbrand's riveting account of the life of Louis Zamperini, a world-class track star who went through hell in World War II and remained *unbroken*.

It was also a personal goal—to remain unbroken.

Fall

When October arrived I was grateful to feel well enough to return to gun, dog, and fields for upland bird hunting, first in Montana and then in South Dakota for the opening of pheasant season. The South Dakota trip was a pilot of sorts for NBC Sports. We wanted to see if there is an audience for a series called *Opening Day*, a tribute to the opening days across the country for events such as walleye season in Minnesota, duck hunting in Arkansas or Louisiana, minor league baseball in the Southeast.

It was a welcome reunion with longtime friends even though my shooting skills were plainly in need of a tune-up. Moreover, walking the uneven ground through thick stands of cornstalks, native brush, and high grass was a wearying experience as it had never been before. My friends all commented on how great I looked but my body reminded me the way back is a long trail.

In November I was invited to join Henry Kissinger

and James Baker, two formidable secretaries of state, on a trip to Berlin, where Baker would receive the Kissinger Prize at the American Academy in Berlin, a study center founded by the late Richard Holbrooke, a passionate student and architect of American foreign policy in Democratic administrations.

Kissinger and Baker reflected on how the West might have handled more effectively relations with Russia following the collapse of the Soviet Union, although they both thought the competing factions in Russia made it very difficult to find common ground.

We were there as Germany was preparing for the twenty-fifth anniversary of the fall of the Berlin wall, which gave me the opportunity to revisit that memorable night in 1989 when NBC News had a worldwide exclusive. I visited the site of my original broadcast, now an entry to a glittering commercial district with luxury hotels, a Porsche dealership, and even a Starbucks. East German students who helped precipitate the revolt are now middle-aged burghers, one with a daughter pursuing a modeling career in Miami.

When NBC News showed video of me that night in 1989 and then cut to me in the same location in 2014 I was startled by my youthful appearance then and the aging Tom Brokaw now. To the audience it was just the passage of time but to me, still struggling with cancer, it was a sharper reminder of mortality.

. . .

Age and news of my cancer seemed to have an effect on organizations responsible for awards. There was the Personal Award at the Peabodys, a coveted journalistic prize. A lifetime achievement award from the National Civil Rights Museum in Memphis. In New York, the Theodore Roosevelt award, named after the cofounder of the American Museum of Natural History, an institution of such surpassing importance scientists from around the world come to study everything from the tiniest vertebrates to the vast mysteries of the cosmos.

At one ceremony I joked that I worried my cancer doctors were sharing with these institutions news they were keeping from me: "He has a limited amount of time left so you'd better hurry." Gratefully, that was not the case.

All awards have their merits but one occupies a special place: the Presidential Medal of Freedom, the highest civilian award in the United States, renewed by John F. Kennedy when he became president. I often joke that one of the unalloyed oxymorons in American life is "humble anchorman," but I was truly humbled when the White House called to say that I had been selected as a 2014 recipient. I hung up the phone and thought of my mother and father, who had their own way of keeping me grounded.

As I began to make my way through various levels of the American success story, Red, as I called Dad, would say, "I always told you, Tom, stick with me and you'll go places." And then we'd both have a big laugh. His other great line, when I was doing *NBC Nightly News*, was "You're doing pretty well but you're no Paul Harvey." He was referring to the very popular Chicago-based radio commentator who had a huge, faithful national following for his conservative views, folksy tales, and distinctive style.

I looked up past recipients of the president's medal, and, sure enough, Paul Harvey was there. Red would be so pleased with the company I was keeping.

Mother's standard line when I was dressed for award events came when I asked how I looked. She'd invariably say, "Nice, dear, but what makes you think everyone will be looking only at you?"

White House aides called with details on the medal ceremony, mentioning that there would be a limit— five—on the number of family members permitted. "No way," I said. "There will be ten guests: Meredith, our daughters, two sons-in-law, and four grandchildren." The limit was lifted.

One of our granddaughters has an aversion to dresses but for this occasion she succumbed to the idea that the White House could be an exception. By train and plane we arrived in the nation's capital and hosted a big party so we could show off the grandkids to longtime Washington friends.

I could hear my mother, Grandma Jean, saying, "My God, Tom, how much is all this costing?" If she had been there I would have put my arm around her, smiled, and whispered, "It's better not to know, Mom."

I've been going in and out of the White House for forty-five years, during times of crises and celebration, and I never fail to get a bit of a rush walking through those corridors taking in the portraits of Franklin Delano Roosevelt, seated at a desk, with that strikingly handsome profile; Abraham Lincoln, his hand cupped at his chin, in the state dining room, looking distracted and exhausted; Jacqueline Kennedy in a long white sheath dress, American royalty; and not too far away, Nancy Reagan, equally elegant in a long red dress.

The honorees and their families were gathered in rooms just off the East Room, where the ceremony would be held after photographs with the president and First Lady. There was a restrained giddiness as old friends and new acquaintances exchanged congratulations and met spouses and grandchildren. I was concerned the Brokaws had excessively topped the limit on guests until Ethel Kennedy came through the door followed by her thundering herd of children and grandchildren.

The Kennedy offspring and ours were friends from skiing and Hyannis Port days in the seventies and now here they were, all grown up with kids of their own.

Vice President Joe Biden bounced into the room and gave special attention to the youngest members of the family, including our granddaughter Charlotte Bird Simon. He leaned over to her and said, "I'll bet you're just as smart as you are cute," a line I'd heard him use before on children but, hey, this was my granddaughter and so it had to be worthy.

As we were summoned name by name—Thomas John Brokaw, Meredith Brokaw, down through the family—for the big photo with President and Mrs. Obama, I teared up as our daughters, their accomplished husbands, and their daughters marched smartly into the setting, poised and yet at ease.

When Michelle Obama gave a hug to the youngest, Claire, the eldest, a San Francisco teenager, said, "Hey, where's my hug?" Michelle laughed and complied.

That same Claire was so at ease as I walked down the aisle into the East Room for the ceremony that she leaned out of her aisle seat and gave me a fist bump as I winked at her sister, another Meredith.

Sitting in the second row, on my right, Isabel Allende, author and niece of the martyred Chilean president Salvador Allende.

To my left, Julia Chaney-Moss, sister of James Chaney, who, along with Andrew Goodman and Michael Schwerner, was brutally murdered in Mississippi in 1964 as they worked to register black voters. I was fully aware of the terrible price their families paid to receive this belated recognition.

As for me, it is not false modesty to attribute this singular honor to my South Dakota working-class roots. As I was coming of age, family, educators, and friends cheered me on when I fulfilled promise and cracked down when I went off the rails. How I wished Mother and Dad were at the back of the room, proud but modest, these enablers of the American Dream. This is for them—and for Meredith, I thought.

It was also a moment for my NBC colleagues who for almost half a century had been there for me. When I returned to New York I sent a memo to the entire news division, citing the role of my personal family but reminding them that they represent my other family.

I wrote them:

The response from all of you to my selection as a recipient of the Presidential Medal of Freedom has been overwhelming and deeply gratifying.

All of you carried me across the goal line more times than I can count—in the studio, on the

*campaign trail, in the flood zones and Cape Ca-
naveral.*

*Triumphs and tragedies. Summits. Tiananmen
Square. Red Square and the Berlin Wall. Nine
Eleven and war, war, war. All of the continents, in
palaces and refugee camps, morning, noon and
night.*

This is your medal as much as it is mine.

Thank you.

Drink up.

As my life was taking a turn for the better I could not
fully enjoy the moment, affected as it was by two upset-
ting developments, each typical of the unexpected cru-
elty of cancer. That young man whom I described as all
but a son to me and a brother to our daughters seemed
to be on the mend from radical surgery to address his
stomach cancer. Mitch, as I like to call him, had written
a poignant letter to friends after his initial surgery.

*I write to you now to let you know I am finally
feeling close to my old self.*

*The last eight weeks really have been a daze.
The will and the stamina to make contact to thank
you just wasn't there. I'm sorry. I was just too worn
out.*

So what did I do all that time? I took it easy. It's

funny. This taking it easy business was kind of
nice. I'd never done it before.
Of course a lot of thinking went on but I will
avoid sharing here "What cancer taught me."
Why?
I don't know yet.

Then, unexpectedly, six months later, he suffered a
mild stroke. He returned to his original oncologist and
received a sobering diagnosis. The cancer was back with
a vengeance. It had metastasized in his lymph nodes, in
several sites within his chest, parts of his abdomen and
sternum. You don't have to be a trained oncologist to
know this is very serious. Systemic, inoperable, and
treatable only by chemotherapy, but first he needs to get
his blood condition back in order.

As I write this he and his family are committed to a
radical gene therapy treatment at the National Institutes
of Health. And our family is committed to helping however we can, which is mostly through the application of
love and prayer.

I received this news as I was staying close to a longtime NBC News colleague whose wife and I were diagnosed with multiple myeloma about the same time. My
friend's wife seemed to be doing well at a New York City
hospital until suddenly, in late 2014, she suffered a

serious stroke and was completely noncommunicative. Slowly, she began to respond and we all had renewed hope. Her husband was, as they say, "cautiously optimistic," until she suffered a severe relapse. He knew what the specialists were telling him: The chances of recovery were gone.

She died the same month Dr. Landau declared my sixteen months of treatment had worked. My blood numbers were back to normal. The chart of the critical markers from September 2013 to January 2015 was a steep, steady decline from the ceiling to the ground floor. I was relieved and grateful for the expert care, hugging Dr. Landau when she finished her presentation, but because of the continuing struggle of friends and the drawn-out death of my friend's wife it was a tempered moment.

Her death, and the emotional pain it brought her husband, was another reminder of Dr. Paul Marks's astute observation that with cancer "medical science has never faced a more inscrutable, more mutable, or more ruthless adversary." For me, it will never again be an abstract condition, something that happens to others. When I read that someone has been diagnosed with cancer or died of it I will know there was nothing routine about his or her experience. The charts showing the improved survival rates for various forms of cancer are instructive, if not always comforting, until the day your physician declares you healed, and even then it is not a money-back guarantee.

My cancer is manageable but remains incurable. However many stories I hear of patients resuming normal lives while keeping multiple myeloma in remission, the numbers, not the anecdotes, tell the hard truths. It's estimated that 24,050 MM cases were diagnosed in 2014, and in the same year 11,090 died of the cancer.

The much more encouraging news is that the five-year survival rate has been improving steadily, from just over 26 percent of MM patients in 1975 to approaching 50 percent now. As the eternal optimist I intend to hang around for longer than five years.

Before he died Louis Zamperini, the hero of *Unbroken*, shared with me the simple recipe for success that got him through his years as a special object of torture and brutality while a prisoner of the Japanese during World War II. "I never gave up," he said, "no matter how hard the beating and torture."

I am not being beaten by a sadistic prison guard. I am subject to the realities of age and the possibilities of recurring cancer or a stroke or a heart attack, but in my mind and in my everyday life I am not thinking, Oh my god, the odds are getting tougher every day.

I want to wake up in the morning with Meredith at

my side, that sunny smile assuring me it will be a good day, not all dependent on the high-profile, jump-on-an-airplane life that had been so routine. Our daughters, their husbands, and now their children provide another narrative rich in its rewards of awe, pride, and laugh-out-loud moments of pure joy.

A marked difference in parenting for our generation is the continuing very close relationship with our children on many levels. When Meredith and I left home we rarely consulted our parents, even though we loved them and respected their judgment. Our lives were sufficiently different about the big decisions—careers, home purchases, child rearing—that we were separated from our parents by changing styles, finances, goals. Now, our children, all in their forties, are constantly in touch about their lives, and I treasure their confidence in us, even when they ignore my advice. It works both ways. They don't hesitate to suggest a new course for me, a subject I am more actively contemplating. There are big ideas to be encouraged, books to be read, museums, films, and theater to attend, river and saltwater flats to be fished, fields to be hunted, fine food and wine to be enjoyed with friends.

If that seems like a mail-order list of clichéd goals, add this: I want more mornings at the seaside in a white terry cloth robe, a large mug of black coffee made with freshly ground beans in a plunge pot or in a filter-lined ceramic cone, Meredith near, reading aloud a quirky item from *The New Yorker* or an email from a grandchild.

Maybe I'll think back to that summer night in 1961 when Meredith and I were sitting on a beach along the Missouri River near our hometown. We'd been seeing each other for nine months, a relationship that surprised her friends and mine. Thanks to Meredith, I was a reformed hell-raiser. She had written me a scathing letter the preceding autumn about my errant ways. I had gone from being a high school whiz kid to being an aimless, hard-drinking, skirt-chasing college student of subpar grades, eventually dropping out.

We'd known and liked each other through high school. She was amused by my ability to twin achievement with roguish behavior.

I admired her discipline, scholarship, and cheerfulness framed by timeless beauty.

When I put my life together after her scolding letter, she apologized for being so harsh and I said, "No, I had it coming." One thing led to another and we were soon dating steadily.

That night on the beach she had recounted how a mutual friend had asked her where this relationship was going and she had answered, "Well, I think we should get married."

I was stunned and momentarily at a loss for words, a rare condition for me.

Really? Yes!

There on the shore of the Missouri River my life took a new direction. More than a half century later I count that occasion as the night my lucky life took a turn that endures to this day because it has been shared with Meredith.

Has cancer changed me? Am I a better person? That's for others to judge. All I know is that in family, access to excellent care, the resources to pay for it, the chance to remain a journalist, and with a cohort of interesting friends, I remain a lucky guy.

So far the early reassurance about my condition is holding up. I will die someday but it is not likely to be the result of multiple myeloma.

I do think about mortality in ways I did not before the diagnosis. It no longer seems a faint, distant reality, in part because I've experienced the ruthless nature of cancer. Simultaneously, at age seventy-five I've moved into the neighborhood of life where there are few long-term leases.

It is not enough to "rage, rage against the dying of the light." It is also a time to quietly savor the advantages of a lucky life and use them to fill every waking moment with emotional and intellectual pursuits worthy of the precious time we have.

Life, what's left.

Bring it on.

Tom Brokaw
Two six four oh

Acknowledgments

I am eternally grateful for the medical expertise, general wisdom, availability, and compassion of each member of my medical team, beginning with Doctors Andrew Majka and Morie Getz at the Mayo Clinic in Rochester, Minnesota; Doctors Heather Landau and Eric Lis at Memorial Sloan Kettering Cancer Center in New York; and Dr. Ken Anderson at Dana-Farber Cancer Institute at Harvard.

My home-grown and very personal physician, Dr. Jennifer Brokaw, was an invaluable member of the team and brought with her large measures of familial love and daughter-father candor.

Our two other daughters, Andrea and Sarah, and our sons-in-law, Allen and Charles, were also part of the extended Team Brokaw.

Steven Brill's personal friendship and his seminal work, *America's Bitter Pill*, first a magazine article and then a book on the complexities, contradictions, irrationalities, and genius of the American healthcare system, were invaluable resources. Another journalist, Frank Lalli, personally went down the multiple myeloma road before I did. His personal experience and editor's eye were beacons for me throughout.

As she has on past book projects, Ruby Shamir turned her

critical research eyes to the many questions about drugs, treatments, types of cancer, and the changing place of hospitals in our daily lives.

At home and in the office, Geri Jansen, Goldine Nicholas, and Mary Casalino were all part of Team Brokaw, keeping me on schedule personally, professionally, and for my medical life. They're uniformly cool, efficient, and resourceful in keeping me vertical and moving forward.

My other family, the men and women of NBC News, were there for me here and abroad, as they always have been. Mike Barnicle and Ann Finucane were there early and often. Stephen Burke, CEO and president of NBCUniversal, generously gave me time to heal and maintain my own work schedule.

This is the seventh book I've written with the encouragement and wise oversight of Kate Medina, my muse, editor, and friend. I wouldn't start another without her. Her encouragement, light but ever-so-effective touch, and friendship were, as they always have been, a tonic during dark days of trying simultaneously to deal with cancer and write about the experience.

Others at Random House include Gina Centrello, Susan Kamil, Tom Perry, Avideh Bashirrad, Benjamin Dreyer, Dennis Ambrose, Evan Camfield, Carolyn Foley, Paolo Pepe, Carole Lowenstein, Theresa Zoro, Sally Marvin, Barbara Fillon, Sanyu Dillon, Leigh Marchant, Erika Seyfried, Anna Pitoniak, and Derrill Hagood.

Finally, a deep bow to all those who know me only as a broadcast journalist and yet took time to write or signal in other ways that they were sending best wishes and hopes for a speedy recovery. As I often say, if there's an oxymoron in my business it is "humble anchorman," but this has been a humbling experience.

ABOUT THE AUTHOR

TOM BROKAW is the author of six bestsellers: *The Greatest Generation, The Greatest Generation Speaks, An Album of Memories, A Long Way from Home, Boom!,* and *The Time of Our Lives*. A native of South Dakota, he graduated from the University of South Dakota with a degree in political science. He began his journalism career in Omaha and Atlanta before joining NBC News in 1966. Brokaw was the White House correspondent for NBC News during Watergate, and from 1976 to 1981 he anchored *Today* on NBC. He was the sole anchor and managing editor of *NBC Nightly News with Tom Brokaw* from 1983 to 2005. In 2008 he anchored *Meet the Press* for nine months following the death of his friend Tim Russert. He continues to report for NBC News, producing long-form documentaries and providing expertise during breaking news events. Brokaw has won every major award in broadcast journalism, including two duPonts, three Peabody Awards, and several Emmys. In 2014, he was awarded the Presidential Medal of Freedom. He lives in New York and Montana.